10403

Skin

Skin

The Human Fabric

By Doug M. Podolsky
and the Editors of U.S.News Books

U.S.NEWS BOOKS   Washington, D.C.

U.S.NEWS BOOKS

THE HUMAN BODY
Skin:
The Human Fabric

Editor/Publisher
Roy B. Pinchot

Series Editor
Judith Gersten

Picture Editor
Leah Bendavid-Val

Book Design
David M. Seager

Art Director
Jack Lanza

Staff Writers: Christopher West Davis,
Kathy E. Goldberg, Karen Jensen,
Michael Kitch, Charles R. Miller,
Doug M. Podolsky, Matthew J. Schudel,
Robert D. Selim, Marcia Silcox

Freelance Writers: Wayne Barrett,
Michael Reinemer

Director of Text Research: William Rust

Chief Researcher: Heléne Goldberg

Text Researchers: Susana Barañano,
Barbara L. Buchman, Laura Chen,
Patricia Madigan, Brenda Mosley,
Ann S. Rosoff, Loraine S. Suskind,
Keith Tanner

Chief Picture Researcher: Jean Shapiro Cantú

Picture Researchers: Ronald M. Davis,
Gregory A. Johnson, Leora Kahn,
David Ross, Lynne Russillo,
JoAnn Tooley

Illustration Researcher: Arthur Whitmore

Art Staff
Martha Anne Scheele, Raymond J. Ferry

Interns: Alicia Ault, John Curry,
Orde F. Kittrie, Jon Lowy, Deborah
Ratner, Harry Zemon

Director of Production: Harold F. Chevalier

Production Coordinator: Diane B. Freed

Production Assistant: Mary Ann Haas

Production Staff
Carol Bashara, Ina Bloomberg,
Barbara M. Clark, Glenna Mickelson,
Sharon Turner

Quality Control Director: Joseph Postilion

Director of Sales: James Brady

Business Planning: Robert Licht

Controller: Elizabeth Humphreyson

Fulfillment Director: Victoria Black

Fulfillment Assistant: Diane Childress

Cover Design: Moonink Communications

Cover Art: Paul Giovanopoulos

Series Consultants

Donald M. Engelman is Molecular Biophysicist and Biochemist at Yale University and a guest Biophysicist at the Brookhaven National Laboratory in New York. A specialist in biological structure, Dr. Engelman has published research in American and European journals. From 1976 to 1980, he was chairman of the Molecular Biology Study Section at the National Institutes of Health.

Stanley Joel Reiser is Associate Professor of Medical History at Harvard Medical School and codirector of the Kennedy Interfaculty Program in Medical Ethics at the University. He is the author of *Medicine and the Reign of Technology* and coeditor of *Ethics in Medicine: Historical Perspectives and Contemporary Concerns.*

Harold C. Slavkin, Professor of Biochemistry at the University of Southern California, directs the Graduate Program in Craniofacial Biology and also serves as Chief of the Laboratory for Developmental Biology in the University's Gerontology Center. His research on the genetic basis of congenital defects of the head and neck has been widely published.

Lewis Thomas is Chancellor of the Memorial Sloan-Kettering Cancer Center in New York City. A member of the National Academy of Sciences, Dr. Thomas has served on advisory councils of the National Institutes of Health. He has written *The Medusa and the Snail* and *The Lives of a Cell,* which received the 1974 National Book Award in Arts and Letters.

Consultants for Skin

John F. Burke is Chief of Trauma Services at Massachusetts General Hospital in Boston and Helen Andrus Benedict Professor of Surgery at the Harvard Medical School. He is a specialist in the treatment of burns and is the co-developer, along with Dr. Ioannis Yannas of M.I.T., of artificial skin for burn victims. Dr. Burke is president-elect of the Surgical Infection Society and a past president of the American Burn Association. Author of more than 200 publications, he is also an editor of a textbook on surgical physiology.

Laurence H. Miller, M.D., is Special Advisor to the Skin Diseases Program of the National Institute of Arthritis, Diabetes, and Digestive and Kidney Diseases, a branch of the National Institutes of Health, in Bethesda, Maryland. He is also on the dermatology faculty of the George Washington University School of Medicine, Washington, D.C., and is engaged in private practice. His special interest in dermatology is the management and treatment of psoriasis. He is the author of numerous articles and papers on dermatology and serves on many medical advisory boards and organizations dealing with skin research.

Ashley Montagu, an anatomist and anthropologist, is well known for his examination of human social and biological evolution. His books, which number more than forty, probe a broad range of topics, including genetics, anatomy and physiology. Among his works are *Growing Young, Touching, The Nature of Human Aggression* and *The Natural Superiority of Women.* Currently a visiting lecturer at Princeton University, Dr. Montagu has also taught at Harvard University and the University of California at Santa Barbara.

Picture Consultants

Amram Cohen is General Surgery Resident at the Walter Reed Army Medical Center in Washington, D.C.

Richard G. Kessel, Professor of Zoology at the University of Iowa, studies cells, tissues and organs with scanning and transmission electron microscopy instruments. He is coauthor of two books on electron microscopy.

U.S.News Books, a division of U.S.News & World Report, Inc.

Copyright © MCMLXXXII
by U.S.News & World Report, Inc.

Library of Congress
Cataloging in Publication Data

Podolsky, Doug M., 1957-
Skin: the human fabric.

(The Human body)
Includes index.
1. Skin. 2. Skin — Diseases. I. U.S. News Books.
II. Title. III. Series.
QP88.5.P63 1982   612'.79   82–12591
ISBN 0–89193–608–4
ISBN 0–89193–638–6 (leather ed.)
ISBN 0–89193–668–8 (school ed.)

20 19 18 17 16 15 14 13 12 11
10 9 8 7 6 5 4 3 2 1

Contents

Introduction:
The Body's Frontier 7

1 The Way of All Flesh 9

2 A Woven Mantle 39

3 Barrier to the World 63

4 Finery on the Fabric 81

5 The Human Touch 111

6 A Thousand Natural Shocks 131

Glossary 156
Illustration Credits 161
Index 162

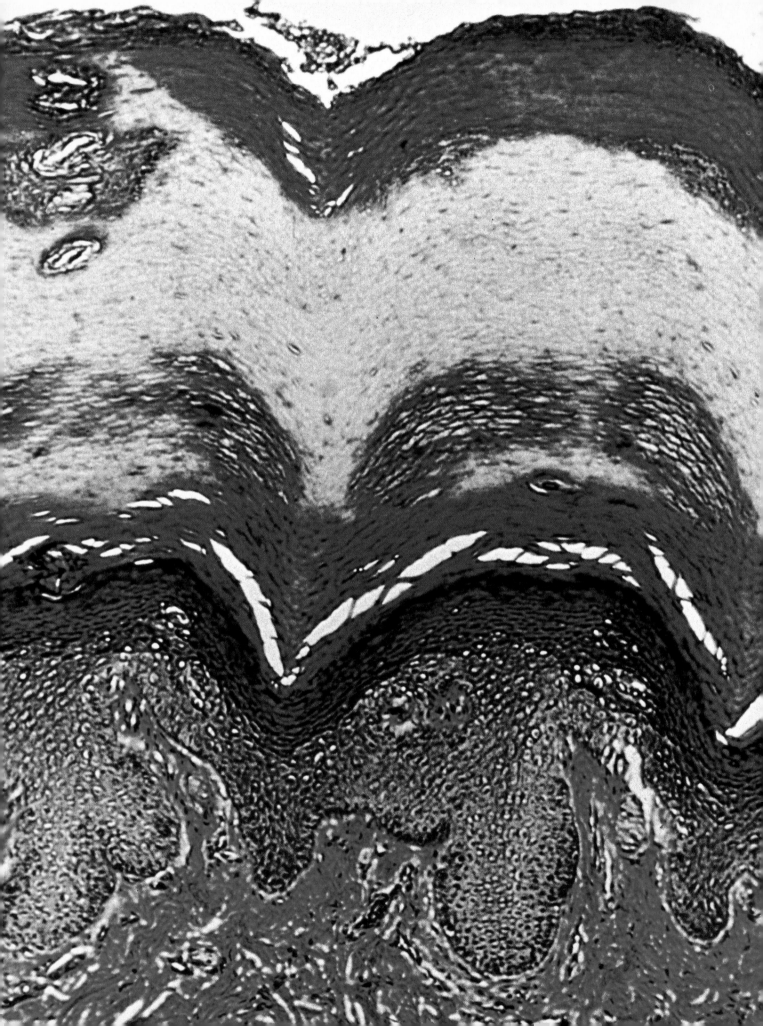

Introduction:

The Body's Frontier

Surely the most visible organ of the body, skin is perhaps the organ most taken for granted, as well. Until two hundred years ago, it was not even considered a system comparable to those of other parts of the body. Silent and immobile, skin registers sensation constantly and supports a teeming, unseen population. It has adapted to its various functions with remarkable versatility. Not only does it harden from use, but it molds into different shapes. As it yields to the most delicate touch, skin becomes an organ of communication, sometimes more eloquent than words.

Knitted together with tough cells, skin protects the soft tissues within the body. Like a frontier of civilization, it is a point of defense, a place at which battles are fought and invaders resisted. Nevertheless, its durable exterior is not an impassable border. By letting water and heat seep through, the skin helps control the body's temperature. Warmth emanating from the skin is a simple measure of our health. Fevers detected by touching the forehead or cheek suggest that an illness has lodged somewhere in the body.

Skin is continually replenished by millions of new cells each day. Resilient as it is, though, it can fail us. It loses its tautness and becomes drier with age. It can be pierced by cuts or charred by fire. Diseases of the skin can lead to death. But medicine is closing in on skin disorders as certainly as it eradicated smallpox, the scourge that condemned millions to death or disfigurement.

Science can conceal imperfections, but through the embellishments of art the skin becomes a tablet for display. Changing cosmetic fashions and hair styles are among mankind's most enduring forms of personal expression. Even if skin is left unadorned, its lines and shading still serve as a record of experience. Skin is our last possession, preserved and valued by us for the character and dignity carried within.

Skin sheathes the body protectively yet lends it sensitivity and feeling. Seen in microscopic cross section here, a fingertip can respond readily to the sudden pang of pain or to the lightest touch of affection. The warmth of human touch led poet Nikki Giovanni to write — without standard punctuation — "i know that touching was and still is and always will be the true revolution."

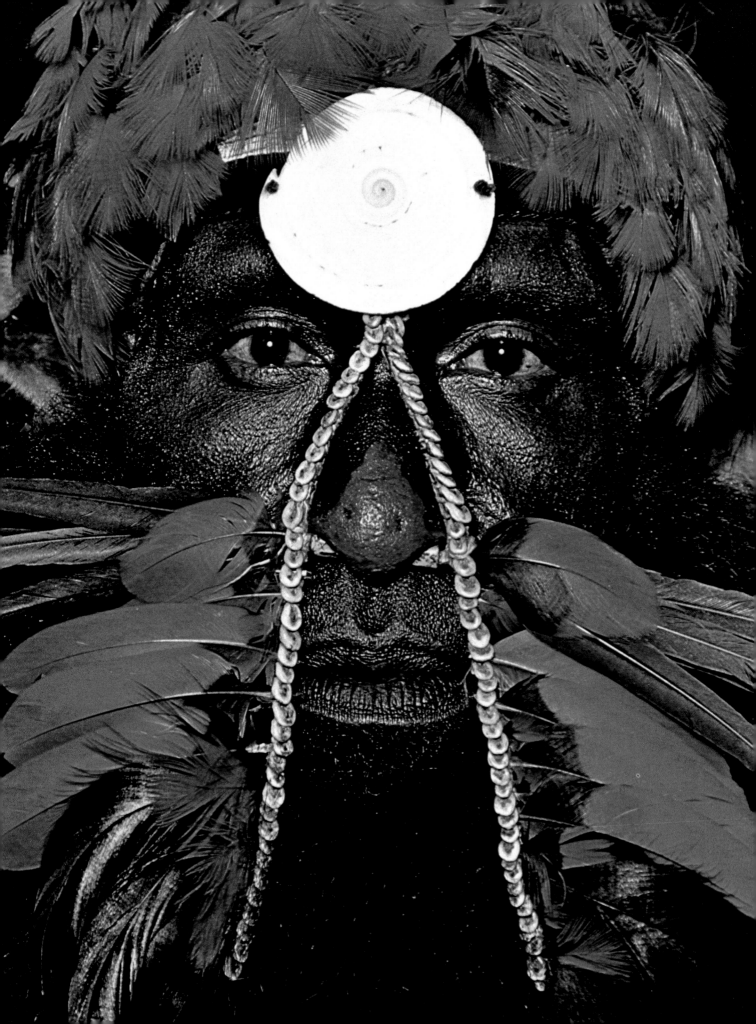

Chapter 1

The Way of All Flesh

Unknown to the West until the 1930s, the people of Mount Hagen in New Guinea practice a complex tradition of body decoration. From whimsical paint enlivening courtship to patterns honoring the solemn relationships with the spiritual world, the body serves as a canvas to dazzle onlookers, stun rivals and aid in everyday business.

S kin for skin," protested Job's tormentor. "All that a man hath will he give for his life." Registering the trials and triumphs of a lifetime, skin is almost universally synonymous with survival. In life and death struggles, the uninvolved lose none off their backs, the lucky escape by the amount on their teeth and victims are flayed alive. Job had lost only his family and fortunes; but, as his ruthless tempter knew, mortal man is tested most when faced with the loss of his own hide.

On our skin, as on a screen, the gamut of life's experiences is projected: emotions surge, annoyances penetrate and beauty finds its depth. Soft, smooth source of youth's vanity, skin later bears wrinkled witness to the toll of years. Radiant in health, it tingles to the affectionate touch. Chilled in the grip of fear, it creeps. Mirroring our body's internal functions, skin's moistness, texture, smell and temperature form physicians' initial diagnoses. From the yellow tinge of jaundice to festering eruptions of smallpox, it is on the skin that diseases make their most disturbing expression. Etched into the fleshy parchment of our palms are the creases of habit that, to the palmist, betray the future. Of age and health, complexions speak frankly, and since the dawn of civilization cosmetics have been sought to amplify or muffle their candor. In the name of vanity and ritual, human skin has endured a host of decorative alterations. From temporary paint to permanent stain, it has been perforated, stretched and geometrically scarred, serving as man's most alluring canvas.

Folklore of many cultures blames man's mortality on matters of skin. A Ch'uan Miao song from China tells of the oldest times when men did not die. As a person grew old, he would simply change his skin like an overcoat and begin a new life. One old woman, her time for changing approaching, instructed her daughter-in-law to

*Embalming alchemy and the oven-
like climate of the Sahara helped
arrest the decay of King Ramses II,
below, who is so well preserved that,
after 3,000 years, signs of arterio-
sclerosis are still apparent.*

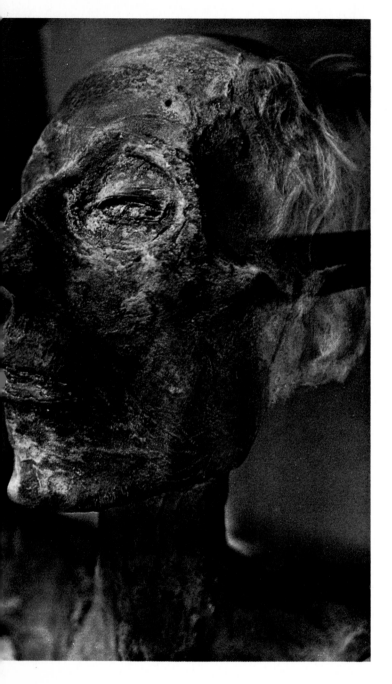

draw a warm bath — the first step of the process.
But the water was too cold, and the old woman
screamed, falling apart in the tub. Her ghost returned to tell the girl: "From this affair death has
come, and it cannot be avoided."

For the Galla tribe of Kenya, immortality was
lost because of a negligent messenger. The god
Wak sent a hornbill to explain to men that when
they felt themselves growing old, they had only
to slough their skins to begin a refreshed exis-
tence. En route to delivering its message, the
hornbill noticed a snake feasting on a carcass.
Thinking of its stomach more than its soul, the
bird traded its message for a portion of the meal.
This is why, the Galla believe, men must die,
while snakes are rejuvenated seasonally.

The shedding snake appears in other legends.
In an Indonesian tale, after God created the
world, he asked all his creatures: "Who is able to
cast off his skin? If anyone can do so, he shall not
die." Because only the snake listened to the offer,
man lost his chance for immortality. The natives
of Banks Island, the westernmost island of the
Arctic Archipelago, believe that at one time man
could change his skin like the snake or crab. One
day, a woman went to the river to cast off her old
skin. When she returned to her child, the infant
screamed and would not accept the new appearance of its mother. Luckily, the skin had snagged
on a branch in the river and the woman was able
to put it back and quiet her child. From that time
on, islanders have grown old and died.

An old slave tale from Guilford County, North
Carolina, tells of two witches who took off their
clothes and skins at night and went out through
the chimney to raid the local store. The store-
keeper sneaked into their house one evening and
sprinkled red pepper on their skins. When they
returned, their skins were too hot to put back on.
"Skinny, don' you know me?" one asked. When
the sun rose, both witches died. From this tale
comes a folk song:

> If I jump in your skin,
> I'll be your popper.
> When you jump out, I jump in,
> An' there'll be you agin.
> You jump out, I jump in.
> I'll be in my skin agin.

Nowhere has skin been linked to mortality with more elaborate ritual than in ancient Egypt. After death, skin decays because of the action of bacteria. This decay can be stopped only by drying, antiseptics or refrigeration. The arid environment of the Sahara provided the first of these conditions. Before the pharaohs, the dead were buried in the hot sands. Losing little more than water, bodies would have undergone a rapid tanning process. Piles of rocks were placed over the shallow graves to prevent jackals and birds of prey from scavenging. If bodies were unearthed, they would have appeared as skeletons covered with skin stretched drum tight — leathery but quite recognizable. Some scholars speculate that it may likely have been this grim spectacle that inspired the Egyptian belief in life after death.

By the reign of Sent, around 4000 B.C., a preserved corpse was considered essential to a contented afterlife. The art of enhancing the desert's drying action approached a peak of perfection three thousand years later. The word "mummy" is derived from the name for a liquid resin used to slow down decay. Natron salts were also widely used. Depending on what one could afford, mummification could take more than seventy days of soaking and marination in palm wine, perfumes, aromatic spices and herbs to a simple pickling in a briny natron bath. With the body's identity ensured, the wandering spirit of the deceased would have no problem finding its way back to its rightful resting place.

The skins of animals have also provided folklore with rich symbolism. Hercules drew his Olympian powers from a lion skin. Adam and Eve were compensated for their fig leaves with animal hides. And Cinderella wore the pelts of ass, cat and mouse to signify her humility. In the Bacchic feasts of ancient Greece, the Maenads, women inspired to ecstatic frenzies, wore panther skins through which Bacchus gave them the power to uproot trees and kill large animals.

The most horrid superstitions were those that inspired believers to practical application. The practices of the Jivaro of the Andean rain forests were among the most infamous. Offering relentless and fierce resistance to the Spanish conquistadors, the Jivaro were the only American Indian

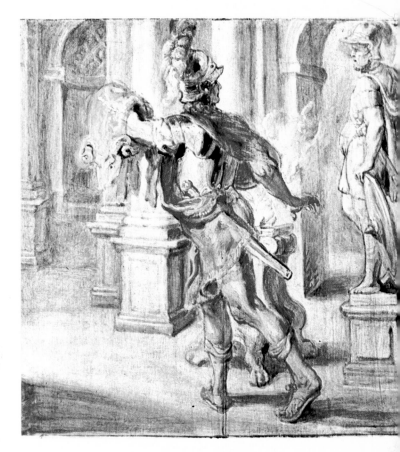

The Golden Fleece of an enchanted flying ram launched one of the most treacherous voyages of ancient mythology. With the return of the fleece, Jason unseated his tyrannical uncle and gained his rightful throne. The hides of such fabulous creatures provide rich symbolism for lore the world over.

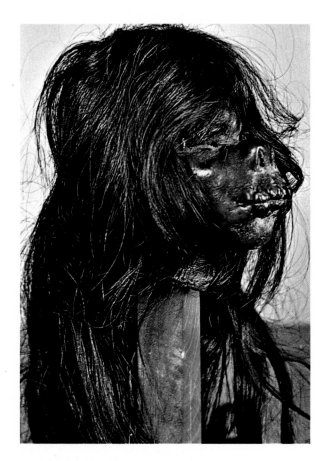

The fist-sized trophy above was once the head of an enemy of a Jivaro of the Andean rain forests. The Jivaro believed that by sewing a victim's eyelids and mouth shut, they trapped his lethal avenging spirit. The skin was painted black to prevent the spirit from peering out and learning the route home. It is said that the Jivaro still practice the technique on the heads of monkeys, which are part of their diet.

tribe ever to overthrow Spanish rule and thwart attempts to retake the gold-rich territory. Much of their success was due to savage methods of taking revenge. By making trophies of enemies' heads, they trapped their victims' *muisaks,* or avenging spirits, and could then chase them away to unfamiliar territory where the spirits would be lost forever. If the head was not taken, the *muisak* could escape the fallen body, pursue the murderer and transform itself into any of three demons: a poisonous snake, a canoe-upsetting water boa or a large tree that would fall on the murderer.

Because heads were cumbersome in fleeing the wrath of a rallied army, the Jivaro would shrink them. They hastily peeled the skin and hair from the skull, throwing the rest into a river as an offering to the anaconda god. The skin and hair were then boiled for half an hour and scraped clean. The eye, nose and mouth openings were sewn shut to form a pouch, which was then filled with progressively smaller hot stones, and eventually hot sand, until the trophy was the size of a fist. The *tsanta,* or shrunken head could then be conveniently carried around the neck. *Tsanta* trophies appeared in curio markets in the late nineteenth century. The Jivaro no longer shrink human heads, but they still practice the ancient technique on the heads of monkeys, which they kill for food.

Some scholars suggest that the Jivaro custom originated as a perversion of a religious rite of the Maya. To honor their deceased rulers, the Maya dried, stuffed and preserved the head skins of their kings in ceremonies. Ancient carvings show attendants playing rattles, flutes and drums and burning incense while priests produce the effigy.

The Skin of Conquest

In the fifth century B.C., Herodotus reported that the ancient Scythians stripped the scalps from the heads of their fallen enemies and sometimes flayed all the skin from their bodies. "Some there are," wrote the Greek historian, "who sew together several of these [scalp] portions of human skin, and convert them into a kind of shepherd's garment . . . this treatment, however, of their enemies' heads is not universal. It is perpetrated only on those whom they most detest."

12

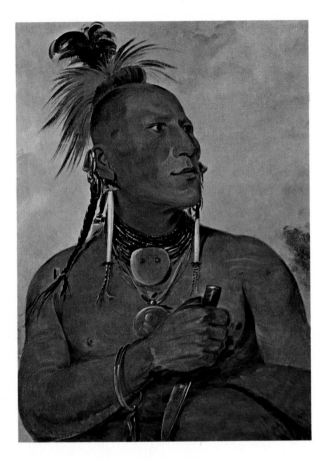

Many North American Indians left a scalp lock on their shaved heads more for utility than for fashion. If a brave fell in battle far from home, his comrades could remove his scalp and carry it home as a token to present to bereaved relatives for funeral ceremonies.

The practice of scalping became all too well known to the early settlers of North America. One of the most vivid accounts of scalping was rendered in a sketch by French explorer Jacques Le Moyne in 1564 that was later developed into an engraving and widely circulated throughout Europe. The Floridian Indians he pictured used razor-sharp reeds to remove scalps. They dried them over fires, and carried the trophies on spears back to the tribe's sorcerer for victory celebrations. Apparently, Le Moyne had not read Herodotus's account of the Scythians, for he declared that it was American Indians who invented the practice. As frontiersmen tried to subdue unfriendly Indian tribes, bounties were paid for scalps from troublesome natives. The bounty system got out of hand in many instances. Aside from cutting scalps in half to increase their remuneration, Indians also unearthed dead bodies for their scalps and raided friendly villages. Despite the brutality of scalping, history has many stories of people who survived the ordeal.

Fur trappers used to tell of a Sioux and a Crow who sat down to play the gambling game known as hands. The Sioux's luck was bad. After losing everything, he bet his scalp and lost. The Crow took his knife, sliced a circle around the Sioux's head and pulled off his scalp with a "sucking pop." The Sioux was silently stoic, asking only for another match. This time luck was with him. His "skull gleaming in the sun and his forehead welted red," the Sioux took everything from his opponent, including his scalp and finally his life. "For years," the story has it, "the Sioux wore both scalps, his enemy's and his own, dangling from his ears."

Early explorers were also shocked by the "grotesque" and "pagan" methods of body decoration they encountered all over the world. While European ladies smeared lead powders and ocher rouges into their faces and forced their figures into hourglass shaped girdles, adventurers were startled by the aberrations of nature they witnessed elsewhere. Whether to be more fierce in battle, more alluring in love, more camouflaged in a hostile environment or more emulative of the wild animals whose powers they sought to invoke, so-called primitive peoples changed the

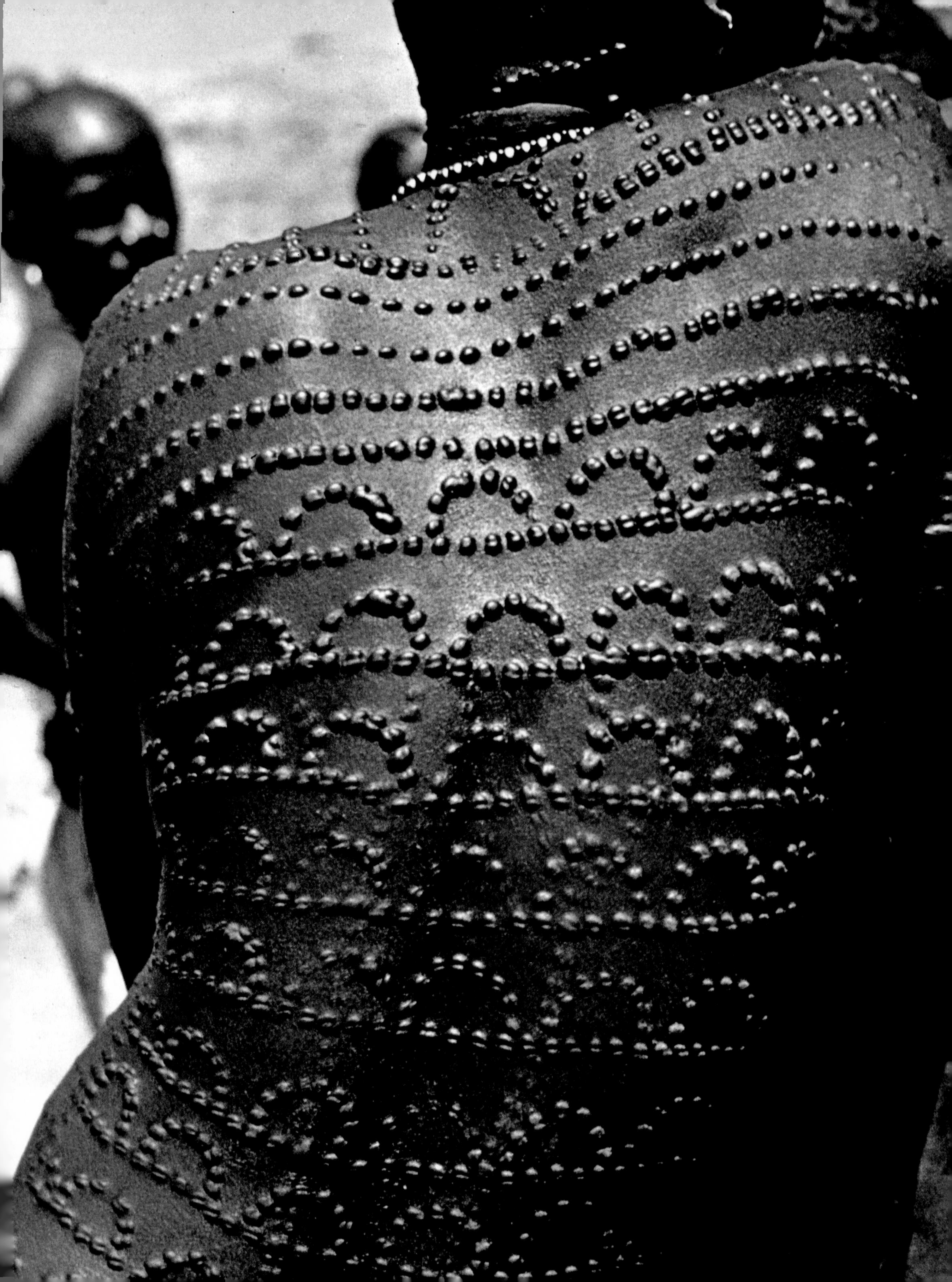

appearance of their bodies to effect a harmony between their spiritual and physical worlds. Paints and dyes were probably their first decorations, but other methods have been used as permanent expressions of their aesthetic values.

Ornamental scarification is most common in Africa. The celebrated masters of the practice are the Tiv of the Benue Valley of Nigeria and the Nuba of southeastern Sudan. The Tiv use razors and nails to make long smooth incisions that conform to the body contours of each individual. Each laceration is immediately treated with a concoction to stop bleeding, then smeared with charcoal or indigo, which makes the scar more pronounced. The pain of the ordeal — arrestingly evident as a swollen lattice of scars — actually enhances the beauty. "Of course it is painful," a Tiv man once told an anthropologist. "What girl would look at a man if his scars had not cost him pain?" With nail and charcoal, a Tiv scarification artist can make a nose appear larger or smaller and accent the play of light on a handsome pair of prominent cheekbones.

The Nuba perform scarification primarily on women. The elaborate patterns of cicatrix, or scar tissue, chronicle the advancement of each girl through the stages of early womanhood. The initial scars come at the first hint of puberty — usually when a girl's breasts begin to develop. The girls are taken to a hillside, the seclusion necessary so that no sorcerers are able to collect the girls' blood. Then, using a hooked thorn to pull pinches of flesh out and a small blade to make crescent-shaped incisions, Nuba women decorate their daughters. A ferric oxide antiseptic is applied. Because of the shape of the incision, extra cells are generated to heal the wound, resulting in shiny, beadlike scars that last a lifetime. In the first stage of scarification, patterns on the stomach signal imminent fertility. The second stage comes when a girl has her first menses. Parallel rows of scars gird her torso just under the breasts. A woman reaches the final stage of beautification when she has finished weaning her first-born child. The back of her body, from midleg to upper neck, is then adorned with more scars. The woman proudly carries the emblems of her rites of passage.

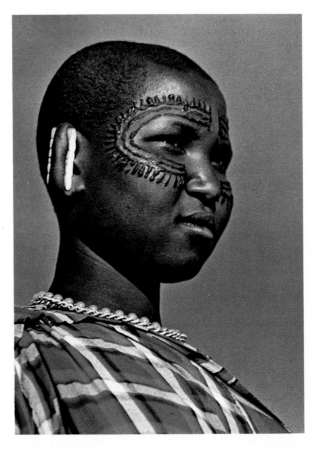

The first two stages of Nuba scarification are paid for with gifts of tobacco or sugar. The final stage, lasting several days, is more expensive. So badly do most Nuba women want the ornamental scars that they often seek out a wealthy lover if their husbands refuse to pay for the procedure. Marriages have been ruined over the matter. When a woman has weaned her first child, she is ready for her final scarring. A matter of vanity and peer pressure, it is also a signal that she is once again sexually available. But there is another incentive. If a Nuba woman dies without proper scarification, it must be performed in the afterlife by a ghostly artist before she can join her ancestors. The work of this artist is said to be more painful than that of any living one.

Whatever the Nuba pay to alter their bodies and conform to accepted ideals of beauty, the costs are easily matched in the West. Each year, 1.5 million Americans spend about $4 billion to

The perforated and stretched earlobe of a Maasai of East Africa, below, serves as a centerpiece for beadwork jewelry. A common custom in much of the area, it is practiced on men and women alike.

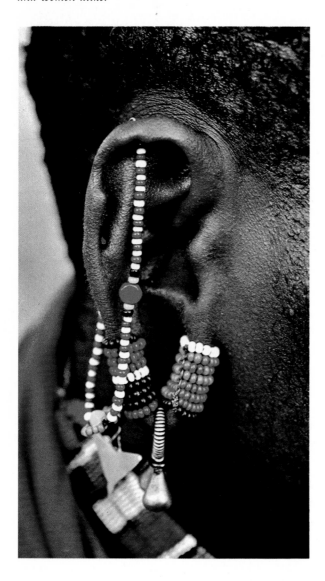

have their noses straightened, chins tucked, breasts enlarged or faces lifted to achieve physical attractiveness in the Western sense.

The Suya of South America exploit another of skin's responsive qualities — its ability to stretch. Puncturing large holes in their lower earlobe, they insert larger and larger disks, until the ears sometimes flop down to the shoulders. The ears are first pierced when a boy reaches puberty. When he reaches manhood, his lower lip is also perforated for a disk. The ornamented disks, after they are outgrown, are considered among a man's most prized possessions. It is also said that Suya men are very embarrassed to be caught without their lip disk, which they take out when bathing. Anthropologist Robert Brain has one theory why only men are allowed to stretch their lips. To the Suya, certain senses are more valued than others. The eye is the medium of witchcraft, evil spirits' entryway into the body. The nose is what animals use to find their way along the ground and, therefore, a lowly organ. But the ear is the sublime instrument of hearing and understanding. Thus, stretching the earlobe improves both. The same principle applies to the mature man's lip. Lectures, orders, judgments and chants are all better delivered through the enlarged lip.

A Pointed Art

In the late 1800s, the two sons of the Prince of Wales went on an extended trip to the Orient. Rumors circulated that both young princes had received elaborate tattoos all over their bodies, including "broad arrows across their princely noses." When they returned, there were, to the disappointment of gossips, no apparent signs of tattooing. On rolling up their sleeves, however, they exposed elaborate dragons on their arms and began a royal fad. Czar Nicholas II, Queen Olga of Greece and King Oscar of Sweden all received tattoos. German Kaiser Wilhelm's chest was emblazoned with a set of "fearsome eagles."

English fascination with tattoos was nothing new. In the first century A.D., Pliny the Elder described the ancient Britons as a people who punctured their skin to form permanent patterns of animals with blue juice from the woad plant. The name "Briton" itself is believed to be derived

16

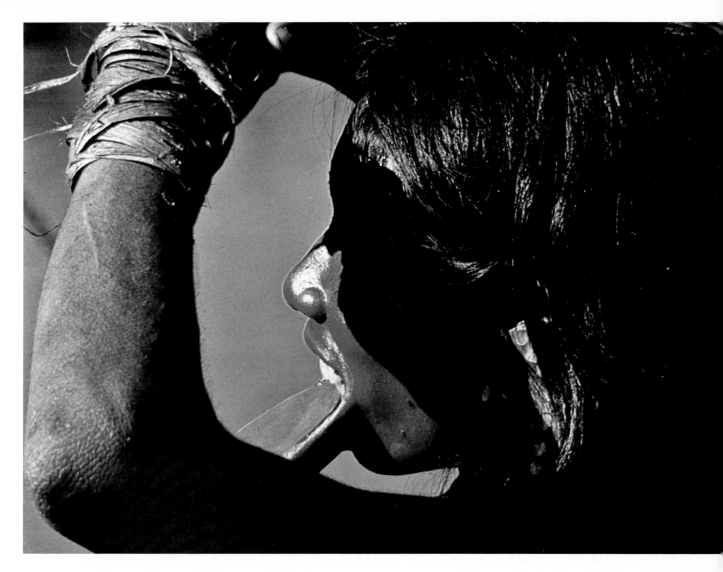

from the Breton word for "painted in various colors." Tattoos have been found on Egyptian mummies, and four stylized birds are tattooed on the hand of an ancient mummy from Peru. In early Greece, slaves and criminals were marked with tattoos for identification. Bone needles and bowls stained with pigment have been recovered from prehistoric caves in Europe.

The Polynesian legend of the origin of tattoos is reminiscent of the Greek myth of Orpheus and Eurydice. A young prince named Mataora married Nuvarahu, a member of the tribe which dwelled in the underworld of Po. After a domestic squabble between the two, Nuvarahu fled back to the underworld. Painting his face for the journey, Mataora descended into Po, where the inhabitants laughed at his feeble facial designs. They wiped the paint off his face and showed him the art of *moko*, which made permanent designs. Mataora rushed back to his home in the

Lip disks, such as the one pictured above, are used by the natives of the Amazon Basin to exaggerate important sense organs. By stretching mouth and ear, they enhance the powers of wisdom and understanding associated with them.

17

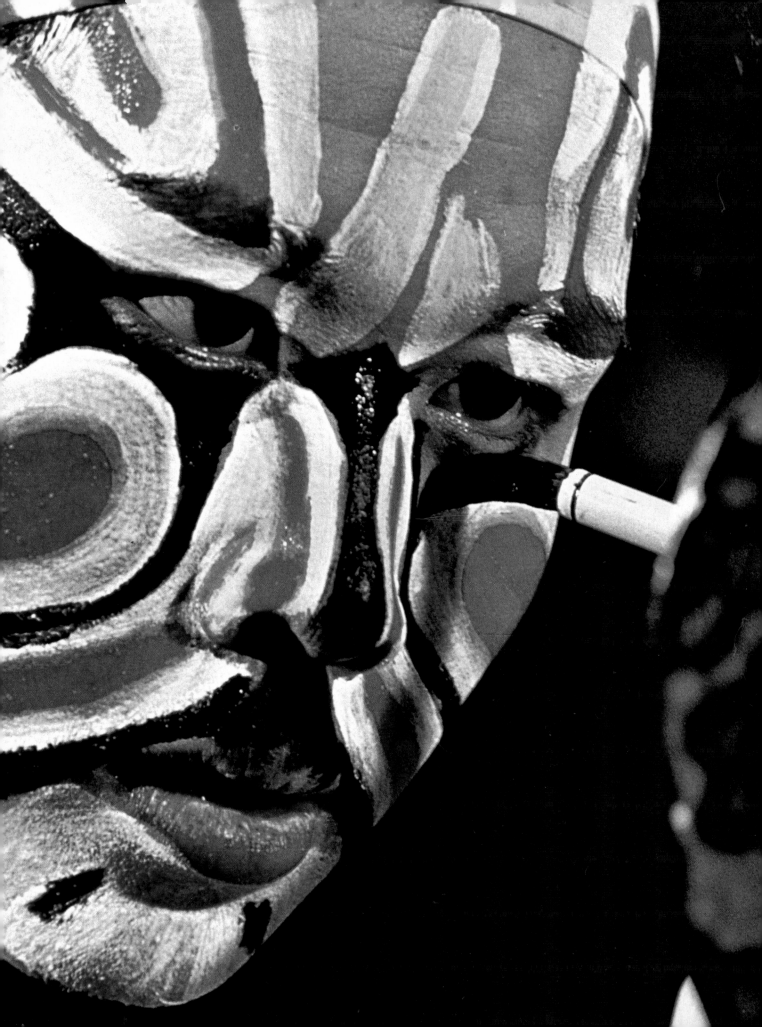

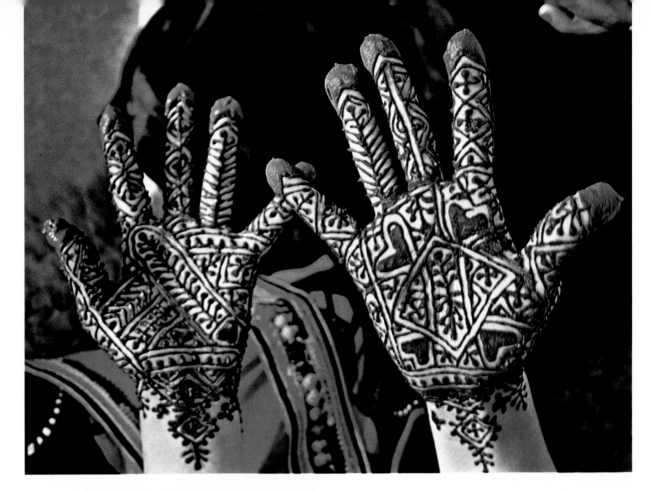

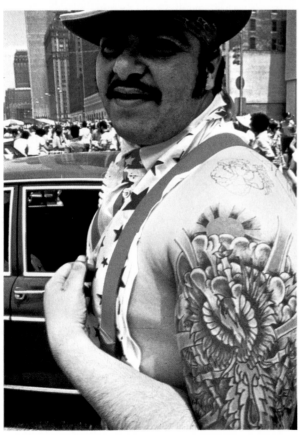

The brilliant make-up of traditional Chinese opera, opposite, originates in primitive religious ceremony. The patterns play upon the art of physiognomy, or face reading, and highlight the traits of stock characters such as the old man, the good man or the rich man. The colors used are also laden with symbolism — red is for goodness and loyalty, white for cunning and resourcefulness, black for honesty, yellow for intelligence. The hands of a Moroccan woman, above, are painted with henna and herb paste not only for beauty but also to protect them during work. In New York City, the Fourth of July is a time for waving banners, including the bold bicep at left.

The elaborate tattoo technique called moko *was perfected by the Maori of New Zealand. Experimenting on slaves, the* moko *artists reserved their finest work for chiefs, below. Conforming to an individual's facial structure, the delicate designs were so admired that the heads were often preserved and put on the auction block. The Japanese art of* irezumi, *tattoos covering most of the body, flourished during the seventeenth century. At right, a fierce Japanese warrior bares his tattooed skin. The dragon — a source of strength and wisdom — and the floral arrangements are traditional* irezumi *subjects still used today.*

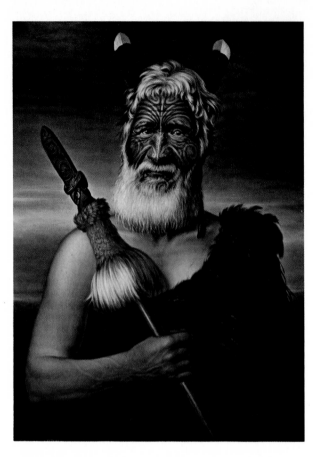

upper world with the new art, but because his wife tried to take a sacred garment along with her, the doors to Po were closed to living men forever. The *moko* system of scratching pigments into the skin that Mataora learned is called *tatau,* from which comes our word "tattoo."

When the young Herman Melville jumped ship in the South Pacific in 1842, he spent a month in hiding among the Typee natives, who practiced *moko* as well as cannibalism. The Typee king and *moko* artist insisted that Melville undergo the body decoration. Tattooing was a religious matter and they were determined to convert the young New Yorker. They could not understand how anyone could object to "so beautifying an operation." Only by repeatedly displaying revulsion at the very thought was Melville able to dissuade the king. The fanciful chronicle of Melville's journey, *Typee,* includes a vivid description of the *tatau* technique.

I beheld a man extended flat upon his back on the ground, and, despite the forced composure of his countenance, it was evident that he was suffering agony. His tormentor bent over him, working away for all the world like a stonecutter with mallet and chisel. In one hand he held a short slender stick, pointed with a shark's tooth, on the upright end of which he tapped with a small hammerlike piece of wood, thus puncturing the skin, and charging it with the coloring matter in which the instrument was dipped. A coconut shell containing this fluid was placed upon the ground. It is prepared by mixing with a vegetable juice the ashes of the "armor," or candlenut, always preserved for the purpose. Beside the savage, and spread out on a piece of soiled tapa, were a great number of curious black-looking little implements of bone and wood.

The technology of tattooing has improved greatly since Melville's time: electric ink-filled needles today prick the skin fifty times per second and are practically painless. But the basic principle of tattooing remains the same. Skin is opened and metal-based pigments are bled in. But why does the body not expel the pigment, as it does splinters and other foreign incursions? The reason is that the pigments used are inert. Cinnabar, cobalt blue, chrome green and mercury red do not react with the body's chemistry. In effect, the body doesn't know they are there. Tattoos are only as irritating as a gold ring on a finger. Without irritation, no rejection reaction is triggered. Normally, lymph cells ingest excessive amounts of the pigment and deposit it in the nearest lymph nodes. Some people, however, have allergies to mercury-based red pigments. In these cases, multicolored tattoos will, over time, lose their red components in an allergic reaction that resembles eczema.

In the 1600s, the technique of tattooing known as *irezumi* began to flourish in Japan. A complete *irezumi* design extends over the whole back, buttocks, thighs and both arms down to the elbows. The painful ordeal costs thousands of dollars and can last a whole year, but to the owners it is well worth it — they have only to disrobe to be well-dressed. *Irezumi* exhibitions and festivals were

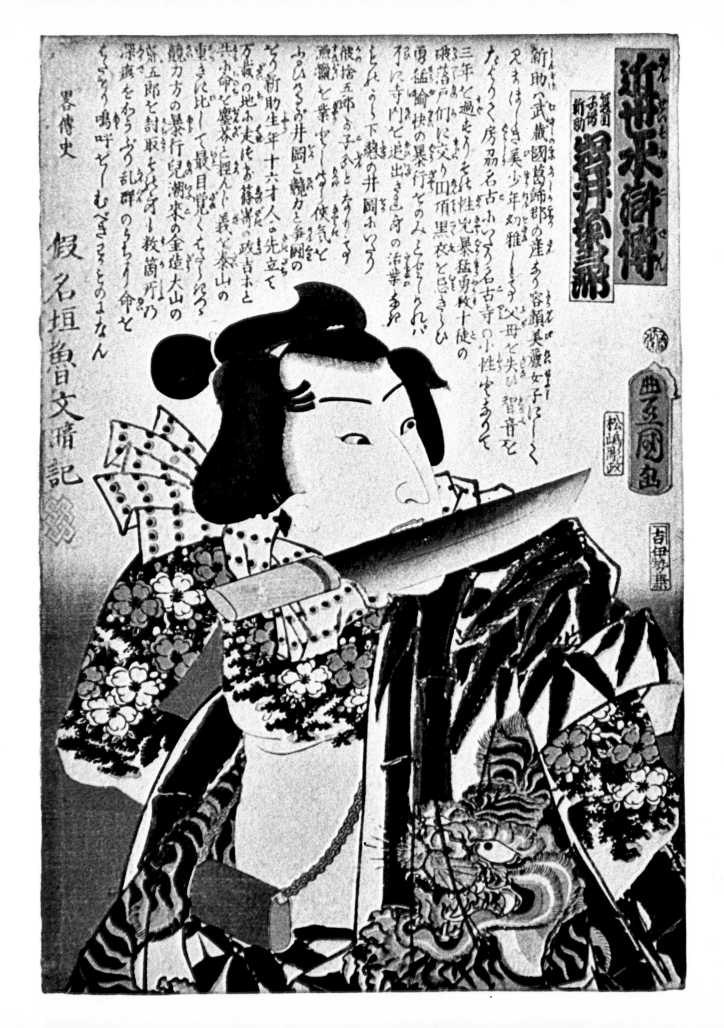

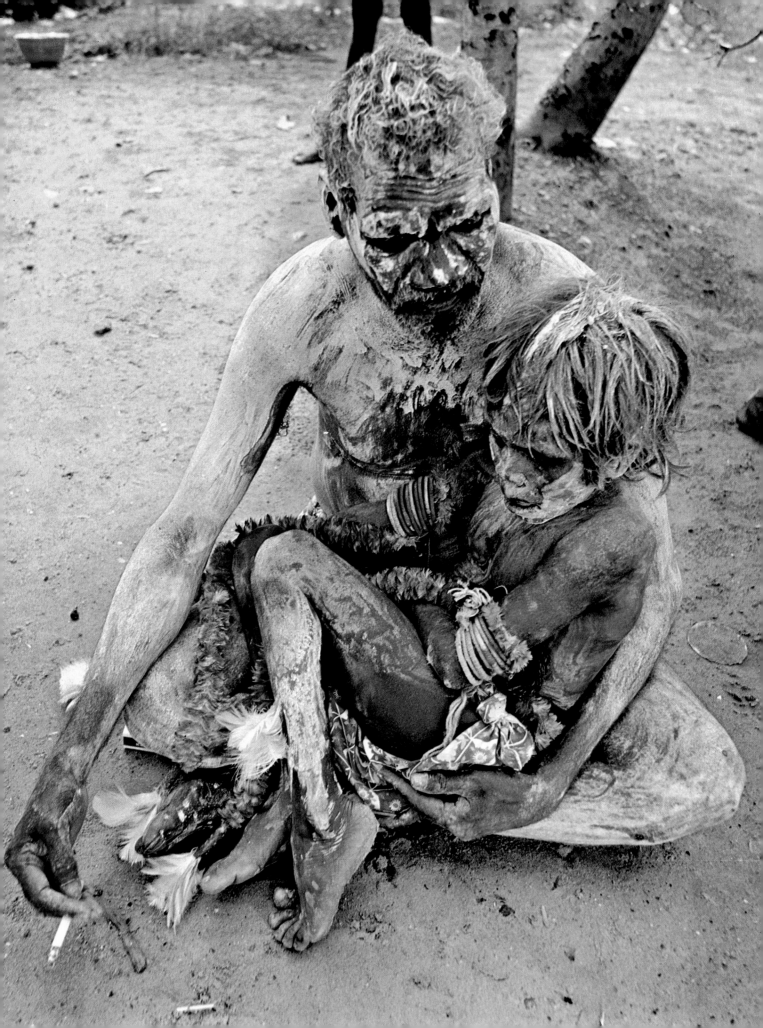

Colors used in body painting have no universal symbolism. At left, Australian aborigines use white paint for mourning and the Hagen of New Guinea, below, use black and white to express aggression.

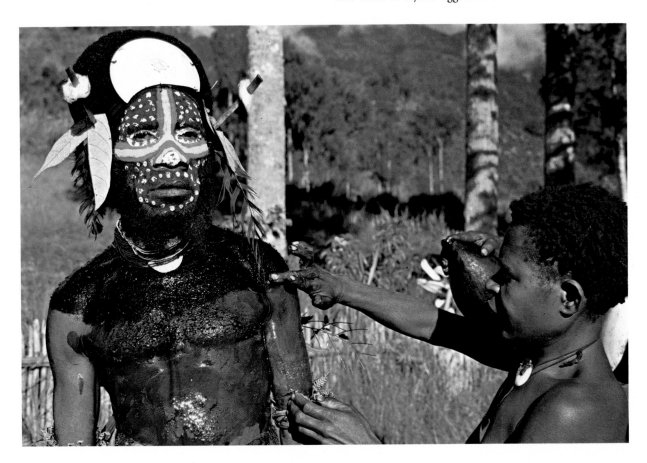

held all over the country in the nineteenth century. Spectacular designs were given awards. Bearers of especially accomplished tattoos received handsome offers to bequeath their hides to posterity. Japanese art galleries and museums still display fine examples of tattooing. The Anatomy Museum of the University of Tokyo Medical School has several *irezumi* mounted for inspection by appointment.

Tattoo owners often regret their adornment and want their tattoos removed. The pigments used today are so physiologically inert that they cannot be coaxed out of the dermis without destroying the skin and forcing it to replace itself. The simplest method is to inflame the skin over the tattoo with caustic chemicals. In the healing process, layers of pigment are sloughed off along with the damaged layers of skin. A new emblem of burn scar remains. Small tattoos can be removed through cryosurgery, or freezing tissue to

death, although it also leaves a scar. With lasers, controlled bursts of beams can be aimed at areas of high pigment concentration, thus minimizing damage to nonpigmented tissue near or within the design.

With a bit of anthropological license, anyone who has ever watched children play with paints can develop a theory of man's first form of body decoration. Body painting is universal. In the name of vanity or superstition, skin, the world over, is rarely left alone. Both color and form take on special significance. For the Australian aborigines, yellow is the color of peace. To mourn the death of a loved one, they smear their bodies with white paint. Natives of New Guinea use black against red paint to celebrate victory in battle or to promote success in trading and commerce. Black symbolizes male aggressiveness, and red is for the warmth, fertility and magic of the feminine mystique.

23

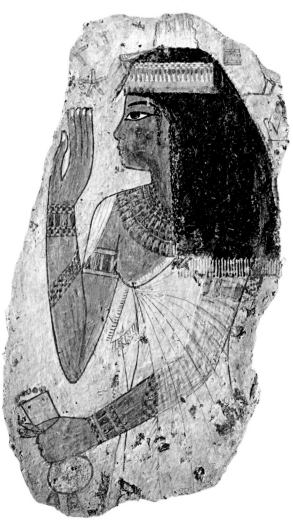

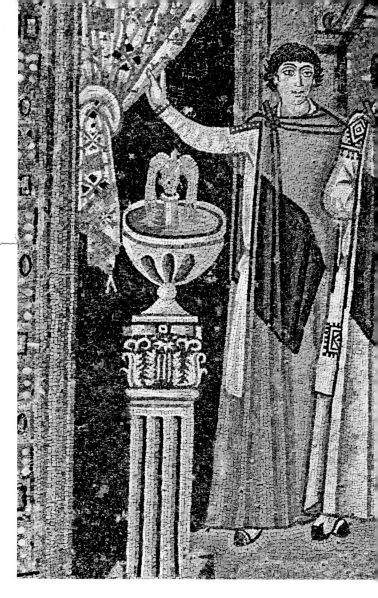

Although the mature mother of an adult son at the time the painting was done, Lady Thepu of Egypt's eighteenth dynasty, above, is represented in the vibrant blossom of her youth. With a perfumed cone in her wig, a seductive diaphanous shawl and a playful wisp of hair over her eye, she captures the ideal of feminine beauty when Egypt was at its height. Cosmetic appliances, such as the golden spoon below, helped women attain the desired look.

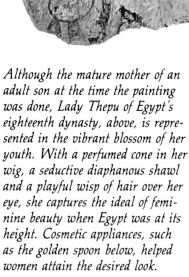

The Thompsen Indians, who lived in the Rocky Mountains, spent their whole winter largely idle, surviving on what they accumulated during the warmer months. In the cold months, they indulged in ceremony, magic and ordeal, using body paint to mark almost every aspect of their lives. Every member of the tribe carried pouches of paint on his belt. "Much of it was for ornament," wrote anthropologist James Teit of the decorations of the Thompsen Indians, "but much also had a strong connection with religion, dreams, guardian spirits, cure of disease, protection, prayers, speech, good luck, war or death." Black circles were painted around the eye sockets as protection against snow or sun blindness, but only by killing an enemy did a warrior earn the right to wear black in battle. Red paint was rubbed into the face and hands to protect skin from the cold, and a red band across a chief's forehead invoked the spirit of the clouds.

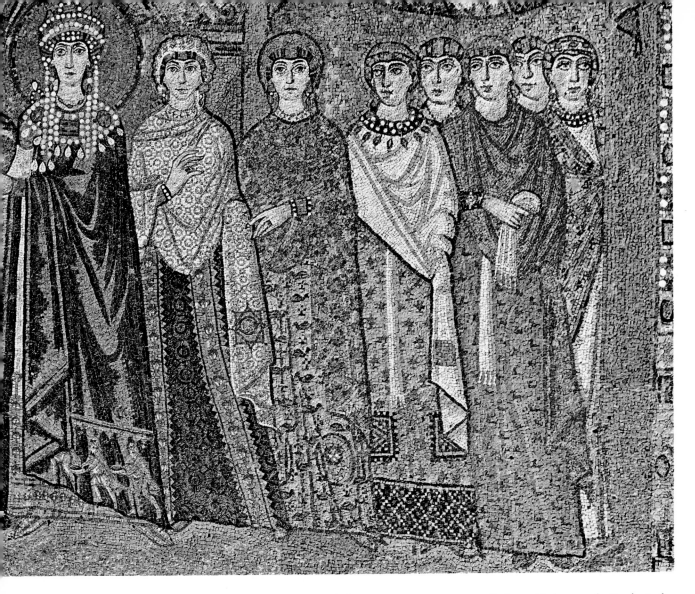

While their women line up to be scarred, Nuba men paint their bodies with designs much more elaborate than those of the Thompsen Indians. Lines of jaw, contours of chin, nose and forehead are integrated into geometrical patterns. The colors and shapes, inspired by animals and birds, vary with different age groups. Each man's role in the community is reflected in his designs.

Throughout these and other cultures, decorative paint alters the appearance of the body and allows people to play the roles assigned by myth, ritual and society. The decorated body — like man himself — mediates between the spiritual world and the rest of nature, creating harmony. It is from the concept of harmony that the Western world derives its word for decorating the body: from the Greek for "well-ordered," *cosmos,* comes our word "cosmetic."

Ancient Egyptians enhanced their natural beauty by outlining their almond-shaped eyes

Posing with her royal attendants for eternity, Empress Theodora gazes from the mosaic tiles of the church of San Vitale in Ravenna, Italy. She began her early life as an actress, married the emperor Justinian and went on to exert influence over the political and religious affairs of the Eastern Roman Empire for two decades. Not a small measure of her allure was attributed to the cosmetic tricks of her boudoir.

25

with kohl, a dark paint. The kohl protected their eyes from harsh sunlight. They applied powdered green copper ore below their eyes, and gray lead ore above them. Women reddened their cheeks and lips with red ocher, stained their palms and nails with henna, darkened their eyebrows with crushed ant eggs and gilded their nipples with gold. Queen Hetepheres traveled to her afterlife generously equipped with an assortment of gold and copper toiletries and more than thirty alabaster jars of cosmetics in her tomb.

The extravagance of the Egyptians held little interest for the Greeks, with their ideals of purity, elegance and proportion. Women might have added a bit of color to their cheeks and lips with red dye from native plants. But it was only the *hetaerae* — women whose livelihoods depended on seduction — who used Egyptian cosmetics.

Roman women, on the other hand, used heavy make-up, inspiring the poet Ovid to warn young men against visiting their mistresses' boudoirs:

> You'll find she's got boxes containing concoctions of all colors of the rainbow, and you'll see the paint trickling down in warm streams onto her breasts. The whole place stinks like Phineus' dinner table, and I've often felt as if I was going to be sick.

Apparently, Ovid did visit boudoirs often enough to form so vivid an opinion. His admonition to women was: "The art that adorns you should be unsuspected."

In order to achieve Ovid's unsuspected look, Roman ladies began each day with a ritual unmatched in ancient times. First, a slave girl, using scented water, would rinse the lady's milk-and-flour night cream from her face. Next, the lady brushed her teeth with a dentifrice of powdered horn, pumice stone and potassium carbonate. A massage with perfumed oils followed a long bath. Unwanted body hair was removed with razors and cream. The lady was then ready for her boudoir. Here, polished silver mirrors, ivory combs, scissors and files, carved boxes and jars awaited her. An *ornatrix*, a specially trained slave, attended her. After her hair was combed, ironed and crimped into shape, her face and arms were dusted with chalk or lead powder, her cheeks

rouged with ocher, lips stained with a dye made from wine dregs, eyes shaded with saffron and powdered ash, lashes darkened with a charred cork and eyebrows neatly plucked.

"Lewde Folyes and Counterfeting"

The Crusades had the most profound effect on the use of cosmetics through the Middle Ages. Among the myriad curiosities brought back from the Orient was the art of face painting. European women began to use make-up to acquire the pale, expressionless appearance considered the ideal of feminine beauty. Many women plucked all hair from their brows, temples and neck to accentuate the oval shape of their faces. Skin creams contained whipped bear's brain, crocodile glands and wolf blood. White lead powder and a hint of rose-red on the lips and cheeks were acceptable, but any further decoration was condemned as idle vanity. This puritanical attitude was expressed in *The Book of the Knight of La Tour Landry,* which warned of the horrors awaiting women who spent hours before the mirror. In one case, the devil changed the reflection in the glass so that one woman saw a sickened visage "so foule and orible" that she never looked in a mirror again or wasted her time on the "lewde folyes and counterfeting" of cosmetics. Since it was believed that women were made in the image of God, they were supposed to be satisfied with their unadorned appearance. Like many inflexible precepts of the Middle Ages, cosmetic habits were transformed by the Renaissance.

Elizabeth I started the vogue for cosmetics in England. She was, as Edmund Spenser wrote, the "Mayden Queen that shone as Titan's Ray in glistring gold and perelesse pretious stone." When she ascended the throne at the age of twenty-five, it was as much her shrewd sense of statecraft as her delicate beauty that captivated her subjects and rallied England's allies. She epitomized the Renaissance. Because her appearance was a political asset, she did not hesitate to turn to cosmetics to preserve it. She drew her make-up devices from Italy, where, according to most reports, the practice had been carried to excess. The poet John Donne no doubt had this cosmetic excess in mind when he wrote:

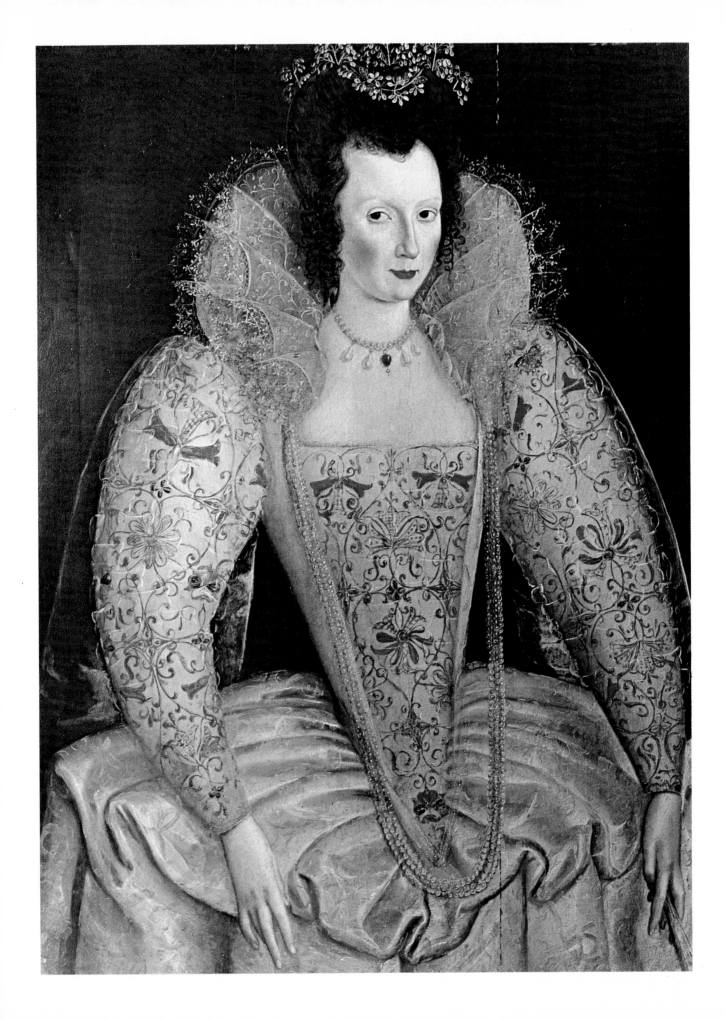

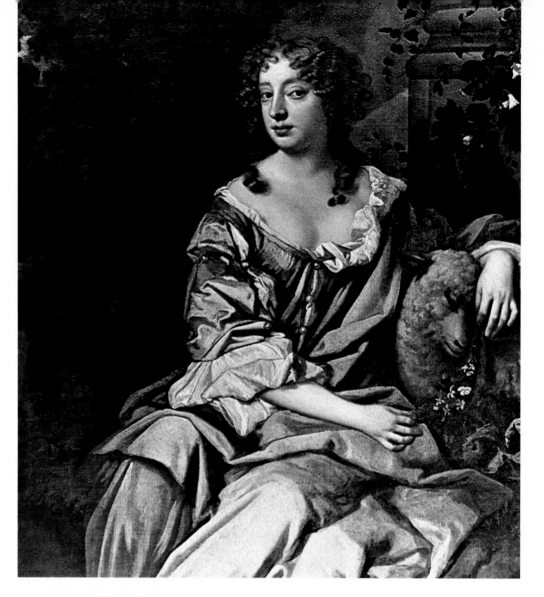

But he who loveliness within
  Hath found, all outward loathes,
For he who colour loves, and skin,
  Loves but their oldest clothes.

Elizabeth's cosmetic practices became the model
for Renaissance English women. The standard
make-up required several steps. White powder
formed the foundation, red ocher blushed the
cheeks, an alabaster crayon painted the lips and a
glaze of egg white preserved the final product. To
guard the complexion against sunshine, both
men and women wore oval masks kept in place
by a button held between the teeth. Make-up
became so widespread that it was discussed on
the stage. "I have heard of your paintings too,"
Hamlet told Ophelia. "God hath given you one
face, and you make yourselves another."

Because Elizabeth had pale white skin, freckles
were thought to mar the ideal of beauty. Sir
Hugh Platt's *Delightes for Ladies* prescribed a cure

for freckles in 1602: "The sap that issueth out of a Birch tree in great abundance . . . doth perfume the same most excellently and maketh the skin very cleer." White wine boiled with rosemary was also considered an effective treatment. Soap was imported from the continent but could also be made at home with cypress, rose leaves, lavender, rosewater and a bit of Spanish soap. Toothpaste consisted of gum jelly and alabaster. Mouthwash was an elaborate mixture of vinegar, rosemary, myrrh, evergreen resin, dragon's herb and fountain water.

In 1603, when the Stuarts came to the English throne, the old argument against "altering God's image" was firmly rebutted with a timely logic. If woman was created in a perfect state of beauty, then what was wrong with trying to overcome the defects brought on by the fall of Adam and Eve? According to a popular ballad, King James I "kept a brace of painted creatures" at his court. Men commonly appeared with fans, perfumed gloves and lovelocks fastened with silk. The cosmetic industry flourished. From Italy came perfumes and cochineal, a brilliant red dye made from pulverizing the dried bodies of female scale insects; India produced yellow turmeric and musk; the Netherlands provided jasmine oils and soap balls; and France supplied orange flower water, apricot creams and Parisian powders. Glass manufacturers fought fiercely over the booming mirror market.

Later in the seventeenth century, cosmetics became even more extravagant. It is believed that the attentions Charles II paid to the comedienne Nell Gwyn inspired women of the day to imitate the exaggerated make-up of the theater. Charles was married to a Portuguese beauty, Catherine of Braganza, whose skin, alas, was unfashionably dark. Faces continued to be whitewashed, cheeks dyed with Spanish rouge and blemishes covered with star- and crescent-shaped patches. Masks were still worn in public. As Charles and his court returned from exile in France, they brought Parisian fashions with them. In 1665, English doctor Thomas Jeamson published the first guide to cosmetic adornment, *Artificial Embellishments, or Art's Best Directions How to Preserve Beauty or Procure It*. As the prices of cosmetics rose, women took to

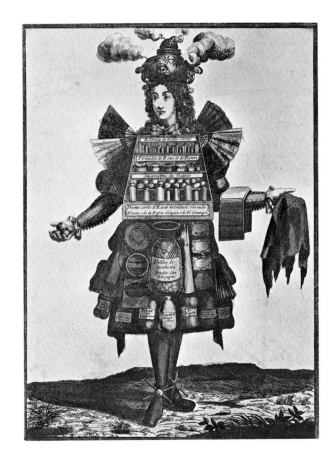

Jasmine oil, apricot creams, orange flower water, turmeric, musk, alabaster toothpaste and Spanish soap balls are but a few of the cosmetic necessities likely available from the seventeenth-century parfumeur, or cosmetic street vendor, above.

29

making their own, often using toxic substances that permanently ruined good looks. Charlatans pushed miracle lotions. The Earl of Rochester, an amateur chemist, posed as a physician and promised a potion that captured the secret of Italy, where women of forty were said to look fifteen. His advertisement said one could "look a horse in the mouth, and a woman in the face . . . and presently know both their ages to a year." He claimed his remedies would not mar the complexion and would rid the skin of "spots, freckles, heats, pimples, and marks of the small-pox."

By the eighteenth century, both men and women in England were wearing make-up daily. Because it was still made of lead, the constant application of such a toxic substance prevented people from keeping their youthful complexions past the age of thirty. Some died from using it. Stylish people also wore false eyebrows made of mouse skin and carried small cork balls inside their mouths to make their cheeks appear fashionably plump. The world of eighteenth-century chic moved poet Alexander Pope to write:

> Such painted Puppets, such a varnish'd
> Race,
> Of hollow Gewgaws, only Dress and
> Face.

In 1770, Parliament acted to protect any man who might be tricked into marriage by the deception of artifice. Any woman found guilty of using scents, cosmetics, false teeth or hair, high heels or iron stays to beguile a man into matrimony would be treated under the law as a witch. The act has never been repealed.

The return, in the early nineteenth century, to tempered, tasteful elegance in Western fashion was largely due to one man — Beau Brummell. Simply rinsing his face every morning with fresh water, he abandoned all cosmetics. Soon, every Regency gentleman in England was imitating Brummell's look of groomed cleanliness. Daily bathing with soap and hot water was recognized as the best aid to beauty and health. Women continued to use cosmetics, but ingredients of herbs, flowers and vegetable oils replaced the toxic substances of earlier times. Blemish removers contained horseradish, sour milk, rainwater,

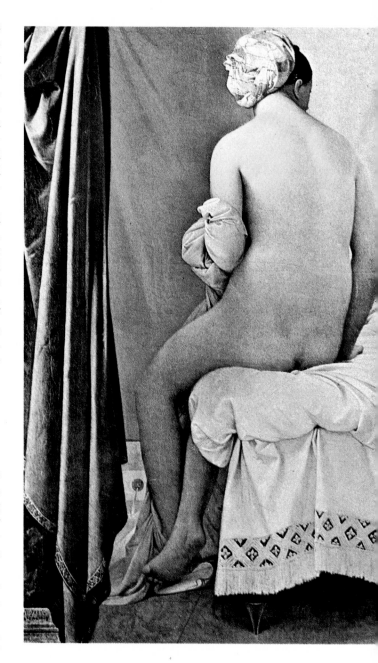

Romanticized above by French painter Jean Auguste Dominique Ingres, the bath was a ritual long ignored through the Middle Ages. By the 1800s, the cosmetic and hygienic benefits of daily bathing were widely recognized.

sugar, lemon and grapes blended together. The Victorian ideal of womanly beauty was an innocent, childlike, untouched look. Cosmetics had to be well disguised. But as the century matured, an image of personality and character replaced the demure style. Women began to imitate the make-up of their favorite actresses — Sarah Bernhardt's carmine lip dye (which, in 1880, she was seen touching up in public), Ellen Terry's dark brows and chalky face and Lillie Langtry's dyed hair. Cosmetic alchemy returned with a fury.

American women now spend over $12.5 billion a year on cosmetics. Dozens of shades and hues are layered and blended to give a "natural look" of wearing no make-up at all. The wrinkle, which never fails to come prematurely, is the greatest target. Nearly $2 billion worth of skin creams were sold in 1980 alone. A single collection of cosmetics could contain several kinds of soap, purifying gels, cellular skin conditioners, astringents, special neck treatments, wrinkle creams specialized for forehead, mouth and eye — all costing hundreds of dollars to replenish throughout the year.

With as much pride as people take in their skin, they are understandably upset when disorders appear. Skin diseases are obtrusive and are much harder to hide than a deepening wrinkle. A very small percentage of people go through life without having some disease of the skin. At any given moment, nearly a third of all Americans have some cutaneous disorder serious enough to warrant a doctor's attention. Because skin disorders are so easily observed, there are many descriptions and fanciful names for skin lesions. Early observations were redescribed and renamed by later generations. Today, dermatologists must identify and treat diseases visible on the skin as well as recognize other diseases within the body that originate in the skin.

In the ancient cultures of the Mediterranean, scanty clothing likely made skin diseases harder to hide and more urgently treated. The diet, hygiene and living conditions probably made skin diseases even more common than they are today. Magic was considered the best remedy. But the regimens often followed in these superstitious rituals were probably scientifically beneficial.

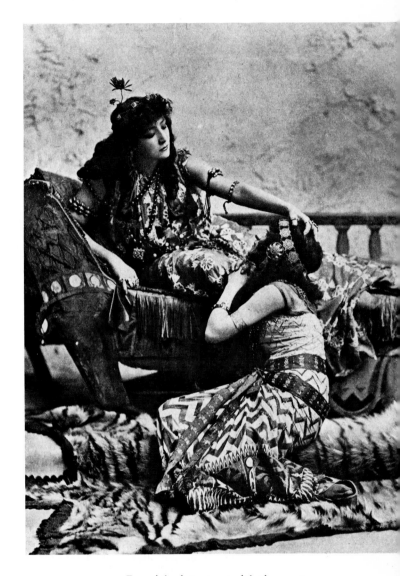

Famed for bringing to life the great tragic heroines of history, Sarah Bernhardt, above playing Cleopatra in an 1890 production, shocked Parisian society by touching up her red lip dye in public. But ladies of fashion soon embraced the taboo shattered by "the Divine Sarah."

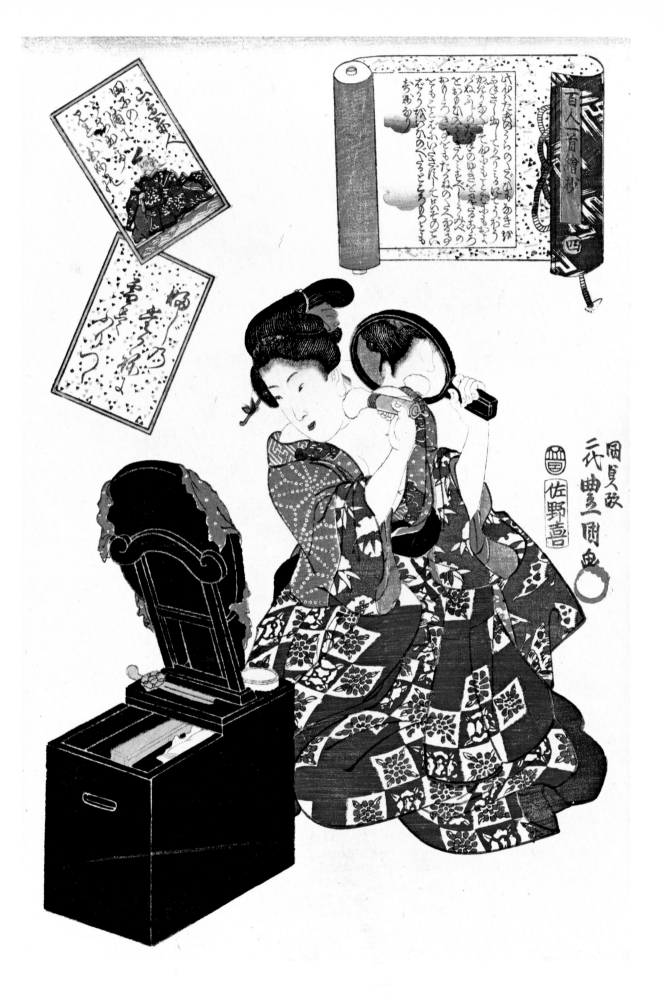

"From Tago no Ura in the distance
I see fresh snow falling on Fuji's
already white crown." So Japanese
poet Yamabe no Akhito describes
the young woman, left, putting
powder on the nape of her neck.

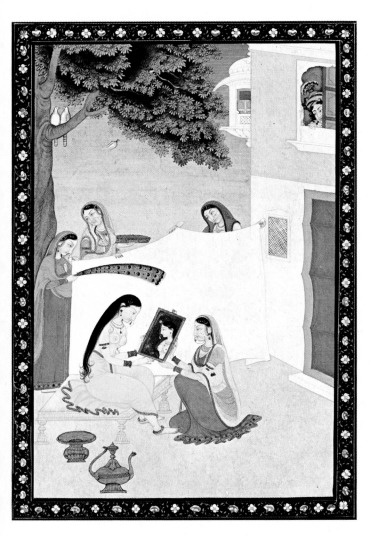

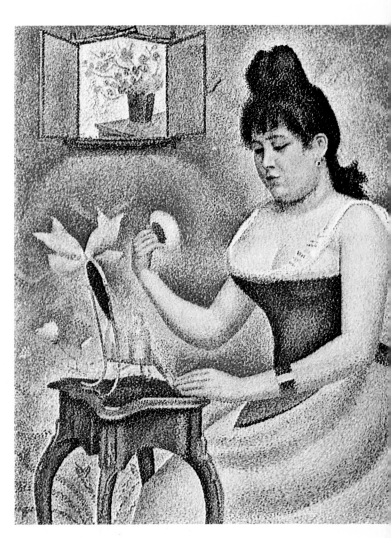

In the nineteenth-century Indian
painting above, handmaidens attend
their mistress Radha in her toilette.
Many of the cosmetic techniques
used by Western women today have
their origins in Asia.

In the heavy bracelets and tight
corset of a traveling player,
French painter Georges Seurat's
mistress, Madeleine Knoblock,
above, poses for her lover in a
gesture of timeless vanity.

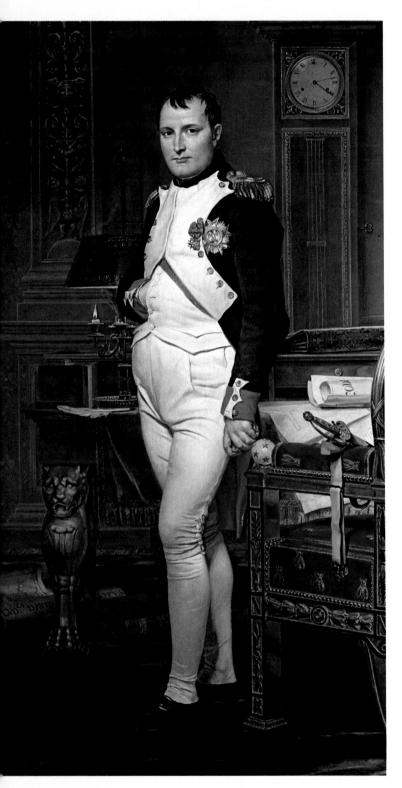

Diets were controlled, exercise and massage were prescribed. Visits were made to the sulfur-rich streams of Syria and the copper deposits of Asia Minor, where the minerals could have helped heal skin lesions. One legendary healing spot that ministered to patients' state of mind was the Temple of Aesculapius.

The son of Apollo, Aesculapius followed in his father's career as physician. It was said that he became so successful at curing illness that he disrupted the immigration of people into Hades. He overstepped his authority, though, when he brought a mortal back to life. As punishment, Zeus struck him down with a bolt of lightning, but Aesculapius survived as the patron god of physicians and medicine. People suffering from skin ailments or disfiguring scars made offerings at his temple. Here, priests would meet them and prescribe appropriate cures. After offering their sacrifice, the pilgrims bathed in the sacred springs and spent the rest of the day exercising or relaxing in the sun. At night, they were led into a lofty bedchamber called the *abaton.* Aesculapius himself often appeared to patients in this room, curing with a divine touch and lecturing on proper health care. Large yellow snakes and dogs, the god's emissaries, wandered freely around the bedchamber and licked the wounds of the ailing. With one touch of a sacred tongue, festering sores would seal, lame legs walk and lush hair sprout on bald pates. These serpents, coiling around a staff, form the traditional symbol of medicine, the caduceus. Carved on the walls of the *abaton* were testimonies from happy customers: "Pandaros had a mole on his forehead. The gods commanded him to place a cloth over the mole and remove it when he left the temple. When he removed the cloth, the mole was gone. But Echenedos, Pandaros's companion, was tricky with the gods about money matters, and instead of removing his mole they gave him another one." Aristophanes, the Greek dramatist of the fifth century B.C., satirized the mythical spa in his play *Plutus.* Aesculapius appears to a blind man and whistles for his snakes, who lick vision back into the man's eyes.

Despite the salt baths and salves, the contribution of classical medicine to our understanding of

34

skin disease was minimal. Hippocrates's system of attributing every sore to an imbalance in the bodily humors retarded the development of scientific treatments for skin diseases. The Roman physician Galen was the first to classify skin diseases according to whether they appeared on the head or over the rest of the body, a distinction that survived till the eighteenth century.

Developing the Language of Skin

Dermatology, like most of the sciences, wallowed through the Middle Ages, supported only by flawed translations and grossly inaccurate summaries of the unquestionable ancients. The catalogue of skin ailments continued to grow. The first real attempt to systematize all known names and symptoms of skin ailments was made in the sixteenth century by Hieronymus Mercurialis, a lecturer at the esteemed University of Padua in Italy. He accepted Galen's classification scheme, but he further divided skin diseases by color, smoothness and thickness. Other physicians soon followed Mercurialis's plan, but many of the resulting catalogues of disease were of little use. Although Mercurialis was a scientist, he was very much a product of his times. He believed that life could spring from decaying matter, but, to his credit, he seriously doubted the popular opinion that lice were created to keep people awake at night so they would finish their work.

With the seventeenth and eighteenth centuries came more and more detailed knowledge of anatomy and physiology. After detailing the workings of capillaries, the great Italian scientist Marcello Malpighi went on to describe the anatomy of skin and sebaceous glands late in the seventeenth century. Soon after, Niels Stenson of Denmark described sweat glands. French physician Jean Astruc unfolded the epidermis, mucous membrane, corium and nerve papillae. Between 1750 and 1825, dermatology grew rapidly as a practical science. Antoine Charles Lorry, the founder of French dermatology, was the first to consider skin a living organ like other systems of the body. He showed that skin diseases often developed from a variety of physiological and environmental causes. The vocabulary available to dermatologists expanded tremendously, bringing new approaches to the diagnosis of skin ailments. The chief pioneer in organizing that language into a manageable grammar was Robert Willan.

Serving for twenty years at London's Public Dispensary for the relief of the sick and poor, he observed a vast array of skin diseases. With precision and clarity, he described each disease at its apex of inflammation. His goal, an understatement of ambition, was to assign a fixed sense to each definition of a skin disease; to classify each by appearance, describing specific forms and varieties; to name and classify all recently discovered diseases; and to specify treatments for all. Willan had accurate color engravings made of each symptom. His greatest accomplishment was the identification and classification of different forms of eczema, a system that holds true today. A heart condition prevented Willan from completing his task, but his student and eventual successor and biographer, Thomas Bateman, did. Willan's work was soon translated into the major languages of Europe. Although many terms he used have changed, the order he brought to the chaos of dermatological study stands as one of the monuments of modern science.

In the meantime, dermatology's first rivalry began to develop across the English Channel. The French Revolution had left an old Parisian plague hospital, *Hôpital Saint-Louis,* in a state of decrepitude that earned it the nickname "sewer of all countries." In 1801, a commission of the National Assembly directed the hospital to take cases of "chronic contagious diseases, scabies, favus, scurvy, ulcers, etc." The world's first dermatological clinic had been founded. J. L. B. Alibert was appointed physician for skin disease at the hospital in 1803 and began lecturing on dermatology. The classification of symptoms became his consuming passion. In 1806, he began to publish a twelve-volume system of dermatology based on his observations at *Saint-Louis.* A witty writer, he described one syphilitic prostitute as a "priestess of Venus wounded by a perfidious arrow of Cupid." He was characteristically French in his observation of minute details, but he frequently made gratuitous generalizations from those details. Although there was little difference in Willan's and Alibert's methods of diagnosis,

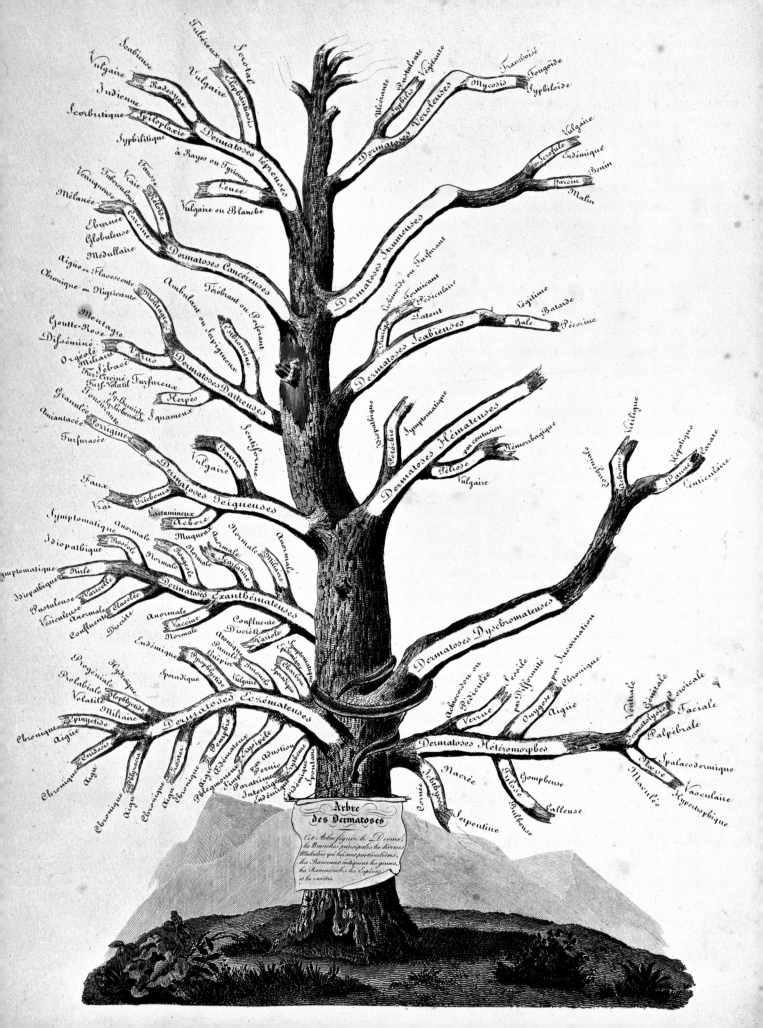

they divided the dermatological world into two camps. Both men tended to overclassify, creating a muddle of redundancies. They also relied too heavily on the external appearance of diseases, grouping together similar symptoms that might have had different causes. Nevertheless, because of their work, dermatology was ready to go beneath the surface.

While Paris and London were the dermatology capitals of Europe, only the most perfunctory treatments were available elsewhere. In Vienna, scabies patients were locked up, visited twice a week by a doctor and given a token arm's-length treatment. On one such visit in 1841, a twenty-five-year-old physician stayed behind to examine a patient more closely. He found something unusual in the shape and color of the sores on the patient's skin. From this simple incident was launched the career of one of dermatology's great masters — Ferdinand von Hebra.

Rejecting the classification of skin diseases by external appearance alone, Hebra approached symptoms from the viewpoint of a pathologist. At a time when the medical world was focusing on the destructive force of microscopic bacteria, Hebra showed how skin could be affected by microbes from without and within. Among the diseases he clarified were scabies, ringworm, rhinoscleroma, impetigo herpetiformis and a form of prurigo, a severe itching disease, that still bears his name. His lectures were the most famous and popular among anatomy students in Vienna. He helped convince the medical world that dermatology was a specialty as worthy of pursuit as surgery or pediatrics. Patients traveled from all over the world to receive his treatments. His students went on to dominate dermatology not only in Europe but throughout the world, carrying with them a principle that still guides dermatologists. "For the recognition of a disease of the skin," Hebra wrote in 1866, "no other assistance is required than a knowledge of the objective symptoms . . . which are appreciable by the sight, the touch, or (sometimes) by the smell . . . they have their origin in the malady itself. They are, so to speak, the alphabet, of which the letters are traced on the skin; and our task is but that of deciphering the writing."

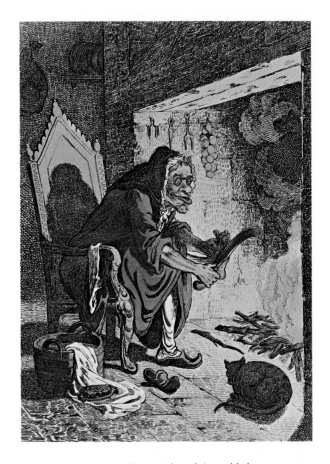

Dermatology has yielded many cures
for age-old ailments. But some, such
as the corn, persist, and desperate
people — like the self-styled surgeon
above — occasionally resort to their
own means of relief.

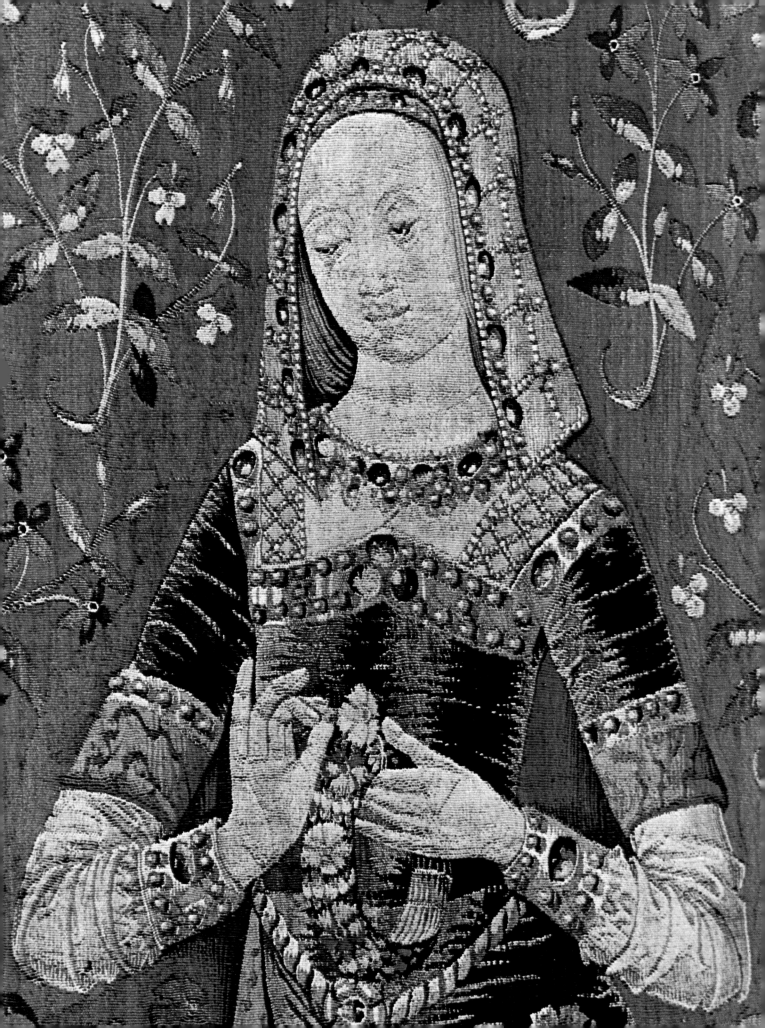

Chapter 2

A Woven Mantle

Skin is an illusory barrier. Dipped by his mother in the charmed waters of the River Styx, Achilles emerged with his skin hardened to armor, save for the heel by which she held him. Only in myth, however, does skin shield man against the harshest slings and arrows of the world. Frontier as well as barrier, skin bounds the body, joining it with and veiling it from its surroundings. It is a lightly defended frontier exposed to the elements with caution and to one's fellows with discretion. American poet Marianne Moore expressed the utter vulnerability of nakedness with three stark lines:

> What is our innocence,
> what is our guilt? All are
> naked, none is safe.

Unlike the stout shell of the armadillo or the rugged rind of the rhinoceros, man's skin is a frontier both open and subtle. Its natural defenses bolstered by care and clothing, human skin readily adapts to extremes of environment. An expanse between twelve and twenty square feet, accounting for 12 percent of the weight of the body, skin harbors touch, the most delicate of senses. Like the basic black dress, skin wears easily on all occasions.

Technically called the integument, the skin is made of three integrated layers — the epidermis, dermis and subcutis — terms that refer to their positions as "overskin," "skin" and "underskin." The outermost layer and immediate buffer to the world outside is the epidermis. The epidermis is the thinnest of the three layers — at most a millimeter, about the thickness of seven pages of this book. Like the other layers, its thickness varies over different parts of the body. Adapted for the everyday friction of gripping and walking, it is thickest on the palms of the hands and soles of the feet and thinnest on the eyelids, which must be light and flexible. The most protean of the

Woven for the betrothed of a French nobleman of the fifteenth century, the tapestry detailed here graced a chateau, telling its tale of a lady and unicorn, a fabled creature popular in medieval times. Skin is a living weave that also spins its own yarns. Furrowed brows, callused hands and scars speak of bygone worries, work and wounds.

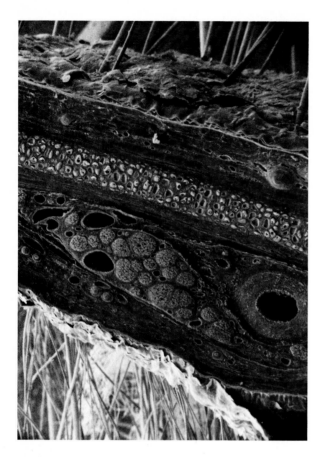

Rich as brocade and sturdy as homespun, skin is a subtle weave. Sectioned, a rabbit's ear reveals its living threads. Hair, stitched through the epidermis and anchored in follicles in the dermis, fringes the fabric. Connective tissue in the dermis lends body to material kept supple by a thick thread of elastic cartilage. Skin takes its touch and finds its feel in bundles of nerves running through the dermis. Tiny vessels coursing with blood lace the dermis to enliven skin's strands. Unlike the finest royal raiments, skin is a cloth of charmed cut, renewing and replenishing itself.

layers, the epidermis also produces fingernails, toenails and hair. In other mammals, claws, horns and hooves grow from this layer.

As in all tissue, the skin's basic unit is the cell. The epidermis is woven of three kinds of cells — keratinocytes, melanocytes and Langerhans cells. Keratinocytes make the protein keratin, cornerstone of outer skin, hair and nails. Melanocytes inject granules of pigment, a coloring agent, into neighboring cells. Melanin, the dark pigment produced, protects the skin by absorbing the sun's ultraviolet radiation. The radiation can damage the genetic structure of skin cells and cause skin cancer. Melanin darkens skin exposed to sunlight. The pigment also accounts for different colors of skin, hair and eyes. Langerhans cells aid the body's immune system by intercepting alien material in the skin.

In the epidermis itself, four distinct layers mesh together to build a hard skin surface. The bottom three layers form the *stratum germinativum,* which produces an armor of tough, dead cells for the fourth, the corneal layer. Sometimes called Malpighian layers, after the seventeenth-century scientist, Marcello Malpighi, who first described them, the *stratum germinativum* consists of basal, spinous and granular layers.

At the bottom of the epidermis lies the basal layer where mitosis, cell division, supplies the epidermis with millions of new cells every day. Because the rate of mitosis depends on the body's available energy supply, the process usually occurs during the four hours after midnight, when other body processes have slacked off. In a cycle that lasts about twenty-seven days, the new cells climb through the epidermis, gradually changing from the soft, columnar cells of the basal layer to the hard, flat cells of the corneal layer from which they eventually slough off. Small attachment plaques called desmosomes bind each cell to its neighbors, so the cells ascend toward the surface of the skin in a continuous, impermeable layer.

New basal cells begin their transformation when they are pushed up into the spinous layer. Here, the cells arrange themselves in vertical columns, and flatten as they move farther up into the granular layer. Granules containing keratin's

Marcello Malpighi

A Scope on Life

Born in 1628, Italian scientist Marcello Malpighi lived in a century of superstition and dogma. Departures from accepted tenets of theology or medicine often met with hostility from authorities in the Church and in academia. The practice of medicine had changed little in 1,500 years. Potions and magic were often considered effective cures.

Malpighi employed the microscope in his study of the body as no one had before. He examined structures of the brain, spleen, kidney, liver, skin and bone that were invisible to the naked eye. After examining a frog's lung in 1661, he wrote that he "could clearly see that the blood is divided and flows through tortuous vessels." Although he did not realize it, Malpighi had discovered capillaries, the final link of the circulatory system. In 1666, he observed red blood cells and proposed that they were the elements that colored blood. He also described taste buds on the tongue, identifying them as the organ of taste, and discovered the dermal papillae, sensitive projections within the skin, as organs of touch. Such was his determination to know the structure of skin tissue that he removed outer layers of his own skin by holding a red-hot iron to it,

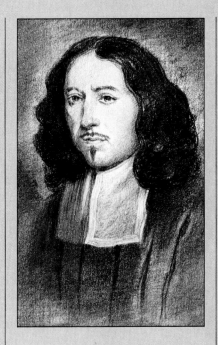

thus revealing the papillae. His discoveries led to future developments in anatomy, physiology and histology, the study of animal tissues.

Malpighi had an insatiable intellectual curiosity. As a youth, he began his studies at the University of Bologna, where he earned doctorates in medicine and philosophy. He later practiced medicine and taught at the universities in Pisa and Messina. The scope of his research ranged widely over the world of living things. He conducted detailed investigations of the chicken embryo. He studied insect anatomy and botany and drew analogies

between the structures of plants and animals. Because of his discoveries, parts of the human body, portions of the insect anatomy and a genus of plants bear his name.

Malpighi drew recognition from home and abroad. He was the first Italian elected an honorary member of the Royal Society of London. Along with his achievements, however, came criticism. Opponents argued that his ideas departed from traditional medicine and that his microscopic observations could not be trusted as accurate descriptions of structures that could not be seen. When he was sixty-one years old, he was actually assaulted by two hostile and, perhaps, jealous colleagues.

Nevertheless, Malpighi received some consolation for his abuse when Pope Innocent XII invited him to be his personal physician in 1691. Malpighi accepted and was further honored in Rome when elected to the College of Doctors of Medicine. He died three years later, but his struggles against the benighted principles of seventeenth-century science were not in vain. For his many accomplishments, he is known as the father of histology, the founder of modern anatomy and botany, and a pioneer of microscopic research.

Tracing trails deep in the dermis,
bundles of collagen pattern the body,
below. Known as Langer's lines,
they correspond closely to creases on
the skin, guiding a surgeon's scalpel
to conceal later scars.

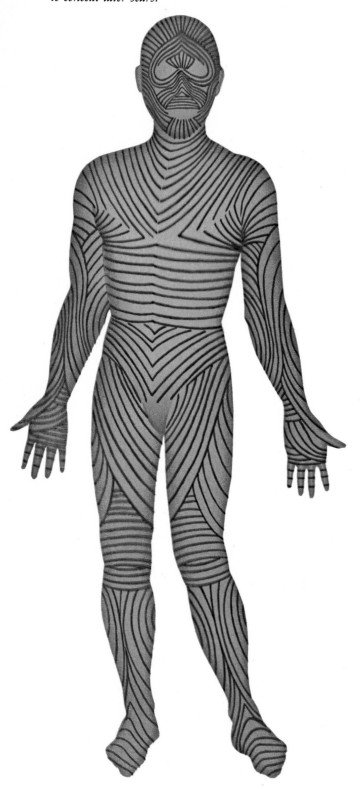

precursor, a preliminary substance, form in the cells when they reach this layer. Then, to become part of the outer coat of skin, the living cells of the Malpighian layers must lose their nuclei and die. Deriving its name from the Latin word for "horn," the corneal layer is made of dead epidermal cells, averaging twenty deep, that create a durable, protective barrier for the layers beneath it. A thin structure called the Reins barrier, resistant to salt and water, further protects living cells from excessive dehydration.

Thick, sturdy and supple, the dermis, or true skin, shields and repairs injured tissue. It also houses nerves, blood vessels as well as sebaceous and sweat glands. Also known as the corium, the dermis is thickest on the palms and soles. This layer consists primarily of collagen. Collagen, originating from special cells called fibroblasts, is one of the strongest proteins found in nature. It gives skin durability and resilience. Certain fibroblasts produce another protein called elastin, related to collagen but more easily stretched. Elastin fibers are especially abundant in the scalp and face, although everywhere in the skin they are far outnumbered by collagen fibers. These two proteins permit the skin to stretch easily, yet quickly regain its shape. They enable the skin to bend and fold with the body's unceasing motions. Collagen also builds scar tissue to heal skin damaged by cuts and abrasions.

Papillary and reticular layers form the upper and lower sections of the dermis. The papillary takes its name from the projections that line the surface of the dermis in mounds or ridges. The papillae carry nerve endings and capillaries, a network of tiny blood vessels, to the living layers of the epidermis. When capillaries rupture, blood leaks into surrounding tissue, giving rise to the black-and-blue discoloration of a bruise. Papillae also supply the epidermis with lymph capillaries to carry away cellular wastes and to aid in removing toxins and dangerous organisms. Visible evidence of the dermal papillae also shows up in skin lines, most notably in the ridges that make fingerprints possible.

Deeper in the dermis lies the reticular layer, where a dense but elastic fabric of collagen fibers provides man's hide. Embedded in this layer, junctions of blood vessels control blood circulation through the skin and so help regulate body temperature and blood pressure. Also packed into this layer are sweat glands, hair follicles and oil-producing sebaceous glands. The collagen bundles of the reticular layer form a pattern known as Langer's lines. In most parts of the body, the pattern follows the skin's crease lines. Surgeons use maps of Langer's lines to guide their incisions in order to disguise or obscure the scars left by their work.

Joined to the bottom of the dermis, subcutaneous tissue is the deepest layer of the skin. Just as keratinocytes produce keratin for the epidermis and fibroblasts produce collagen, the key element of the dermis, lipocytes make lipids, fat globules, for the subcutaneous tissue. This fatty layer cushions muscles, bones and internal organs against shocks. It also acts as an insulator and stores energy against lean times.

Like the hard cells of the corneal layer, hair grows from the living layer of the epidermis. The hair root, reaching deep into the subcutaneous tissue, rises from a special structure, the follicle. Taking its name from the Latin word for "little bag," the follicle is a thin sac of epidermal tissue with a bulb at the bottom.

Adjacent to the hair follicle, connected by a short duct, are two or more sebaceous glands that provide oil for the hair and outer skin. These glands produce sebum, a mixture of waxes, fatty acids, cholesterol and debris of dead cells. Unique to mammals, sebum coats both hair and fur with a waterproof shield that helps insulate the body from the rain and cold. Since man has lost all but a few patches of hair and has clothed and sheltered himself against the elements, he no longer needs much sebum for insulation. But his glands still produce it in abundance.

Aside from enhancing the insulating properties of hair, sebum serves several other functions. By coating the dead keratin cells of the corneal layer and the hair, sebum sequesters moisture, keeping hair glossy and skin pliable. Sebum also contains a precursor of vitamin D that produces the mature vitamin when struck by the ultraviolet rays of the sun. Sebum may also kill certain forms of harmful bacteria.

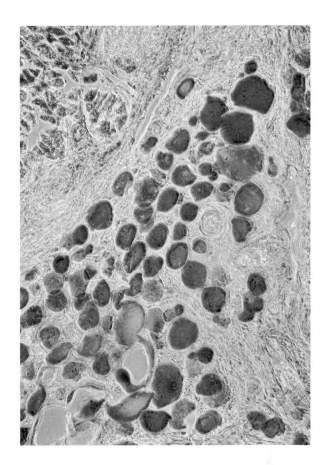

Fat cells, like these in a knee, fill subcutaneous tissue, the innermost layer of skin. A cache of energy, fat cells are consumed when nutrients run short in the blood stream. The last line of skin's defenses, subcutaneous tissue cushions muscles, bones and organs against shocks while shielding the body from cold.

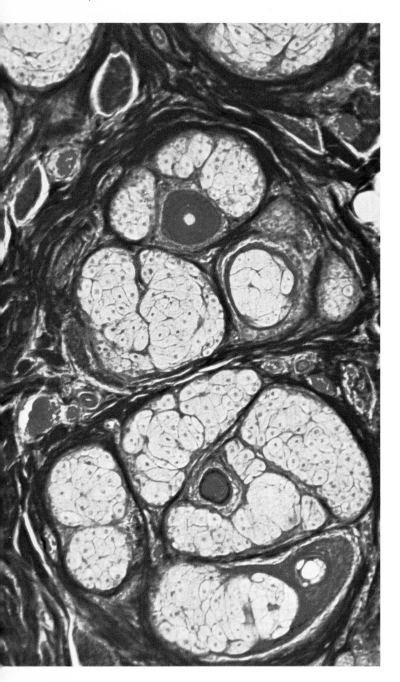

Cells crowd closely within sebaceous glands lying alongside hair follicles. Filled with fats, these cells secrete sebum, a waxy mixture produced only by mammals, to lubricate and protect skin and hair.

Sebum takes many forms — earwax, dandruff and the crusty matter that collects around the eyes during sleep. Sebum gathers on the face and scalp, where there are proportionately large numbers of the glands. Sebaceous glands coat the skin continuously, more copiously in men than in women, owing to the effect of the hormone testosterone. Occasionally, the glands supply too much sebum. This condition, called seborrhea, gives the hair and skin a greasy sheen. Even with a normal rate of sebum production and regular washing, the sebaceous glands and hair follicles of the face, neck and upper back create conditions favorable to acne, perhaps the most common disorder of the skin.

A Pall Over Man

Virtually everyone experiences acne. It may linger long after adolescence or afflict adults for the first time in their twenties or thirties but, usually, acne occurs during teen-age years. The ancient Greeks knew that acne accompanies the advent of puberty, but it was not until the nineteenth century that scientists associated it with sebum and hair follicles. During puberty, hormonal changes in the body spur the sebaceous glands to activity. Researchers have identified testosterone, a hormone produced by both men and women, as the specific trigger. A heightened production of sebum increases the likelihood of acne. Other factors may cause or compound the condition, such as genetic inheritance, bacterial growth, emotional stress, changes in climate, certain cosmetics and environmental conditions. Although no particular foods have been found to cause acne, diet is widely thought to contribute to it. Chocolate, long a prime suspect, has been exonerated by recent research.

Acne begins in the hair follicle. Normally, dead keratin cells produced by the follicle lining are carried to the skin's surface but, occasionally, they fall apart and stick to the lining. The cellular debris forms a plug, or comedo, at the opening. Bacteria living in the follicle produce an enzyme that breaks down sebum into free fatty acids. These acids irritate the lining and eventually cause the follicle to burst, releasing the sebum and acids into the dermis. The ruptured follicle

Most common during puberty when hormones increase the flow of sebum, acne arises as dead cells fail to clear a follicle. Bacteria in the adjacent sebaceous glands produce enzymes to turn trapped sebum to fatty acids.

The acids first irritate then burst the follicle. Acids and sebum spill into the dermis, inflaming the skin and causing a lesion. Lesions may appear on the surface of the skin as pimples or deeper, as cysts.

inflames the skin and forms a lesion. In the most common form of acne, acne vulgaris, the lesions form blackheads, named for the dark appearance of melanin in the comedo, and pimples. Cysts, larger lesions in the skin, characterize the more serious cystic acne.

Acne has long cast a pall over man. Marcellus of Bordeaux, court physician to fourth-century Roman emperor Theodosius, recommended that a person wipe the skin with a cloth at the instant a shooting star crossed the sky. In the eighteenth century, some physicians advised marriage as a cure in the belief that masturbation sparked acne, an idea that lingered into this century. Recent research has brightened the outlook for chronic sufferers for whom a broad range of treatment is available. Antibiotics like tetracycline, erythromycin and clindamycin are commonly used to destroy the bacteria in follicles. Dermatologists also administer the female hormone estrogen, which reduces sebum production. The treatment is usually restricted to female patients because of the feminizing influence of the hormone on males. Vitamin A acid and benzoyl peroxide help by stimulating mitosis in epidermal cells, thus hastening the release of the follicle plug. Other treatments include drying and peeling agents containing sulfur, sunbathing and, in rare cases of cystic acne, X-ray treatment. The most promising new development is a derivative of vitamin A called 13-cis retinoic acid, which has shown remarkable success in curing cystic acne, apparently by reducing sebum production. Because cystic acne frequently leaves scars, this treatment buoys hope that lasting damage can be avoided.

Acne scars can be removed or at least obscured by dermabrasion, a refined technique of cosmetically smoothing the skin first practiced by the ancient Egyptians. One Egyptian remedy prescribed applying a paste of alabaster particles suspended in grain, honey and milk to the face. In modern dermabrasion, facial skin is anesthetized and frozen at −30° C for fifteen to thirty seconds while a dermatologist smoothes the tissue with a spinning diamond wheel. Treatment can be completed in twenty minutes. Although the skin takes weeks to heal, dermabrasion can effect a striking change in appearance.

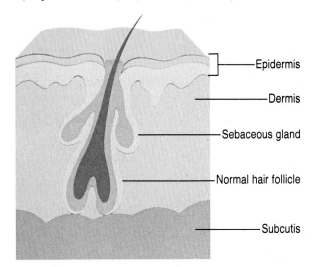

Epidermis

Dermis

Sebaceous gland

Normal hair follicle

Subcutis

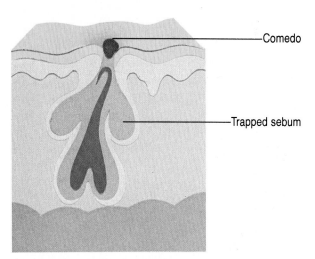

Comedo

Trapped sebum

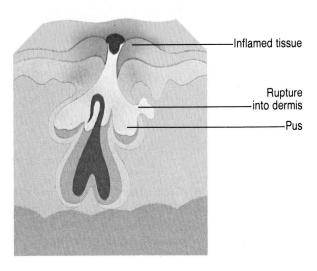

Inflamed tissue

Rupture into dermis

Pus

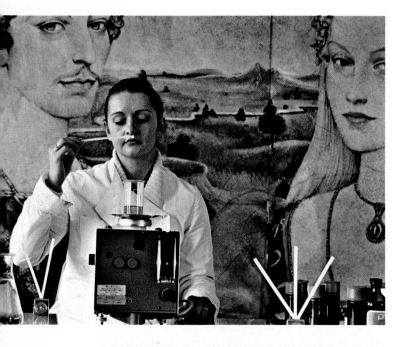

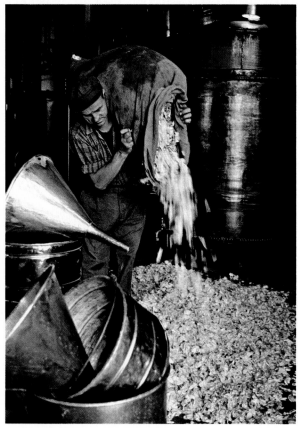

In his quest for beauty, twentieth-century man has shown great ingenuity in devising means to alter his physical features. Plastic surgeons can restore injured or malformed parts of the body by molding skin tissue and bone. The same surgical procedures are often used to alter the body for purely cosmetic purposes. Wrinkled or sagging skin can be easily tautened anew.

Man has also found fault with another natural process of the skin, sweating. In seeking ways to suppress it, he has attempted to overcome a biological necessity. Throughout human history, sweat has represented a universal symbol of toil. In a soliloquy, Shakespeare's Hamlet asks why, but for the fear of death, would man "grunt and sweat under a weary life?" In a tight spot, we break out in a "cold sweat." And although we do not actually "sweat" blood, the body does produce different sweat through two mechanisms, the apocrine and the eccrine.

The apocrine glands become active during sexual maturation and are therefore considered a sexual characteristic. They respond not to heat but to the excitement of fear, anger, sexual arousal or other strong feelings. Immediately responding to the emotions, the glands secrete a small amount of cloudy fluid, squeezed out by a muscular sheath. Like the sebaceous glands, they open into the hair follicle to gain access to the skin. Apocrine glands are found only in the armpits, the ear canals, the nipples and around the genitals. The female breast is an apocrine gland that has evolved to perform a different function.

In other mammals, apocrine glands produce pheromones, scents that serve social functions. Human apocrine glands may be the vestigial remains of a once prominent scent system in man that also played some role in social behavior, perhaps producing an aphrodisiac or a territorial marker. In the fetus, during the fifth month, rudimentary apocrine glands appear over most of the body but disappear within a few weeks. So many fetal apocrine glands suggest that man once had a much greater need for them.

Apocrine glands still play a role in social behavior, but a negative one. In pure form, apocrine sweat has very little odor. But when bacteria that normally live on the skin feed on apocrine sweat, it acquires a smell. General aversion to body odor has long sustained the manufacture of perfumes and deodorants. Perfumes have been used for thousands of years to sweeten the scent of the body. Now, with antibacterial agents and chemical antiperspirants, man can suppress his natural scent for short spells. Ironically, some perfume makers use musk, a glandular secretion of the male musk deer, in an effort to elicit residual instinctual responses that may still exist in men and women.

The Sweat of the Brow

The sweat that dampens the brow comes from eccrine glands. Numbering between two and three million, they produce much more sweat than apocrine glands. Eccrine glands can secrete as much as three gallons a day in hot weather. Excessively salty sweat from the eccrine glands is a unique and reliable sign of cystic fibrosis, a lethal hereditary disorder of the exocrine system. Doctors encourage mothers to kiss their children often; the salt is readily tasted.

As a thermoregulator, the eccrine system reacts to signals from the hypothalamus in the brain by moistening the skin. The sweat, almost all water, evaporates on the skin and draws excess heat out of the body, maintaining constant internal temperature. Certain eccrine glands respond to other stimuli. Glands in the forehead, underarms, palms and soles work at times of psychological stress, independent of heat or exertion.

As with apocrine glands, fetal development hints at the evolutionary significance of the divided eccrine functions. At three-and-a-half months, the fetus has glands on the palms and soles. Eccrine glands do not develop on other parts of the body until the fifth month. One biologist suggests that early man needed moist palms and soles to strengthen his grip and lighten his touch when threatened.

Another feature of the hand and foot that evolved for both gripping and locomotion are the papillary ridges. Labyrinthine lines that trace distinctive, revealing patterns, the papillary ridges most commonly appear as fingerprints. These ridges, covering the palm and sole, run counter to the direction of gripping motion. The lines follow

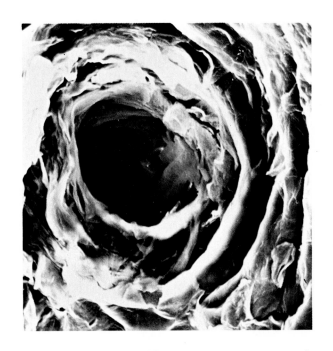

Highly sensitive to temperature and temperament alike, between two and three million eccrine glands perspire in response to heat, effort and stress. They may release as much as three gallons of sweat on a hot day. Under stress, the glands dampen the forehead, armpits, palms and soles.

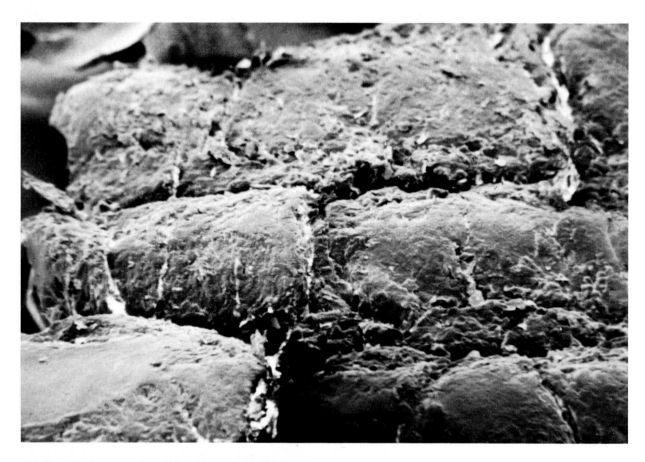

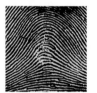

When highly magnified, the skin covering the fingertips loses its familiar appearance. Rounded ridges rise above shadowed valleys. The terrain of all fingers follows contours of arches, loops and whorls, shown left to right. Yet close scrutiny of the number and arrangement of ridges within these patterns reveals infinite variety. No two individuals, living or dead — not even identical twins — possess one and the same set of fingerprints.

the deeper pattern of the dermal papillae that push upward into the epidermal layers. Apart from enhancing grip, the ridges provide more skin area for cell regeneration than a flat surface would allow. The ridges develop a permanent pattern during the third and fourth months of fetal development. No two individuals, even identical twins, have the same fingerprints.

A Printer's Art

Dermatoglyphics, the study of fingerprints, separates fingerprints into three basic patterns — arches, loops and whorls. The lines of an arch run from one side of the finger to the other with an upward curve in the center. In a loop pattern, the lines begin on one side, loop around the center and return to the same side. The lines of a whorl form a circular pattern. Each of these patterns has variations. For precise classification, a fingerprint technician looks at two key formations, the core

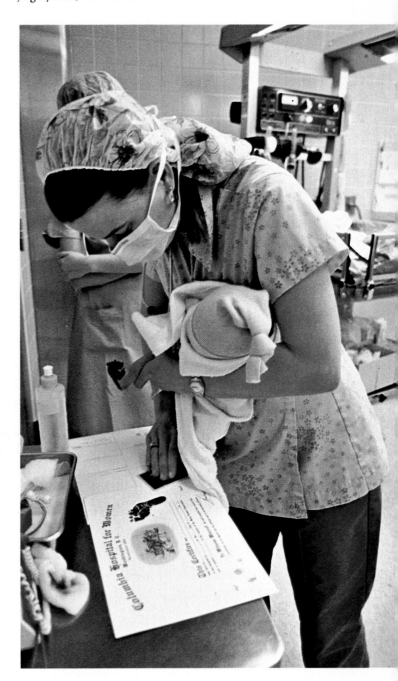

Born into the world innocent but anonymous, babies exchange their prints for identity in the delivery room. Because babies live hand to mouth, footprints, rather than fingerprints, are recorded.

and the delta, to count the number of ridges. The core is the center of a loop or whorl, while a delta marks the divergence, the splitting of ridges near the core. For loop patterns, the ridge count is reckoned by counting the ridges touched or crossed by an imaginary straight line drawn from the delta to the core. For whorls, the ridge count indicates the number of ridges touched or crossed by a straight line between two deltas near the core. Since deltas and cores are not identified in the arch pattern, the ridge count for an arch is always zero. Once a fingerprint is assigned a type and a precise ridge count, it becomes easier to differentiate among others. The pattern of eccrine pores along the ridges is another feature that permits more detailed comparison of fingerprints. The number and arrangement varies from person to person.

In each individual, the right hand pattern differs substantially from the left. Between men and women and among different peoples, fingerprint patterns occur in different frequencies. Although sex cannot be determined by fingerprints alone, women tend to have more arch patterns than men, while men tend to have wider skin ridges.

In newborn babies, unusual ridge patterns can signal abnormal development. "Accidentals," unusual patterns that do not fit within standard classifications, occur more frequently in congenitally abnormal babies whose mothers contracted German measles during pregnancy.

Prints have long been used to establish the identity of individuals. Hospitals routinely footprint babies at birth. A small skin area is all that is needed to identify accident victims who are otherwise unrecognizable. Occasionally, fingerprints have been used to restore identity to amnesia victims. Fingerprints are now used in civil service and academic tests. As early as the seventh century, the Chinese applied fingerprints to legal documents, a ceremonial practice that confirmed the authenticity of the agreement.

By far the oldest and most common application of prints has been in the solution of crimes. In first-century Rome, palm prints figured heavily in a murder trial. Legal scholar Marcus Fabius Quintilianus proved a blind boy innocent of killing his father by establishing that bloody hand

49

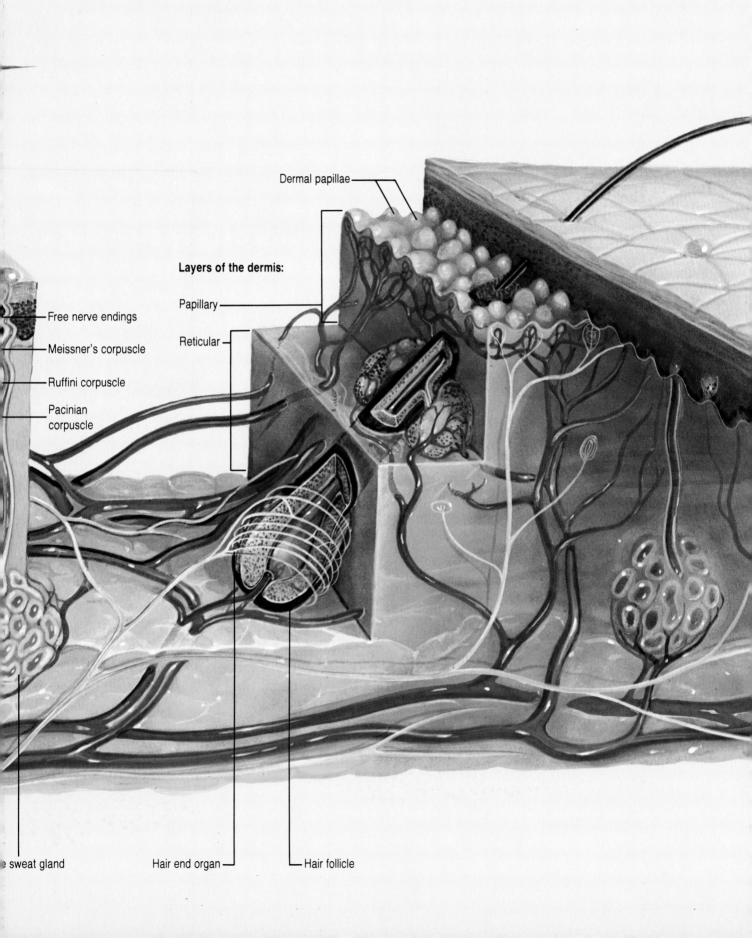

Dermal papillae

Layers of the dermis:

Papillary

Reticular

Free nerve endings

Meissner's corpuscle

Ruffini corpuscle

Pacinian corpuscle

e sweat gland

Hair end organ

Hair follicle

THE MULTILAYERED SKIN

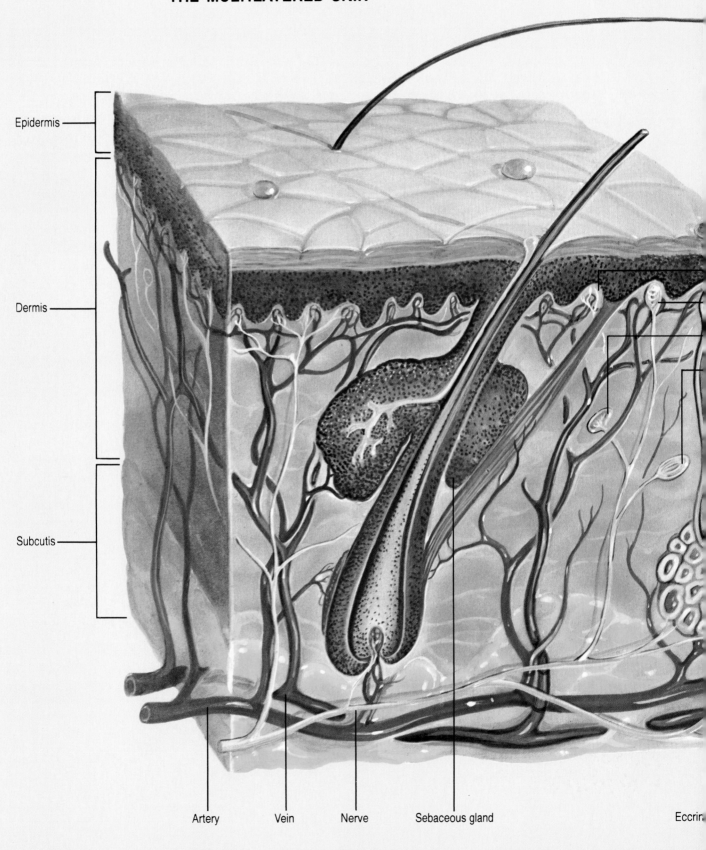

Epidermis

Dermis

Subcutis

Artery   Vein   Nerve   Sebaceous gland   Eccrin

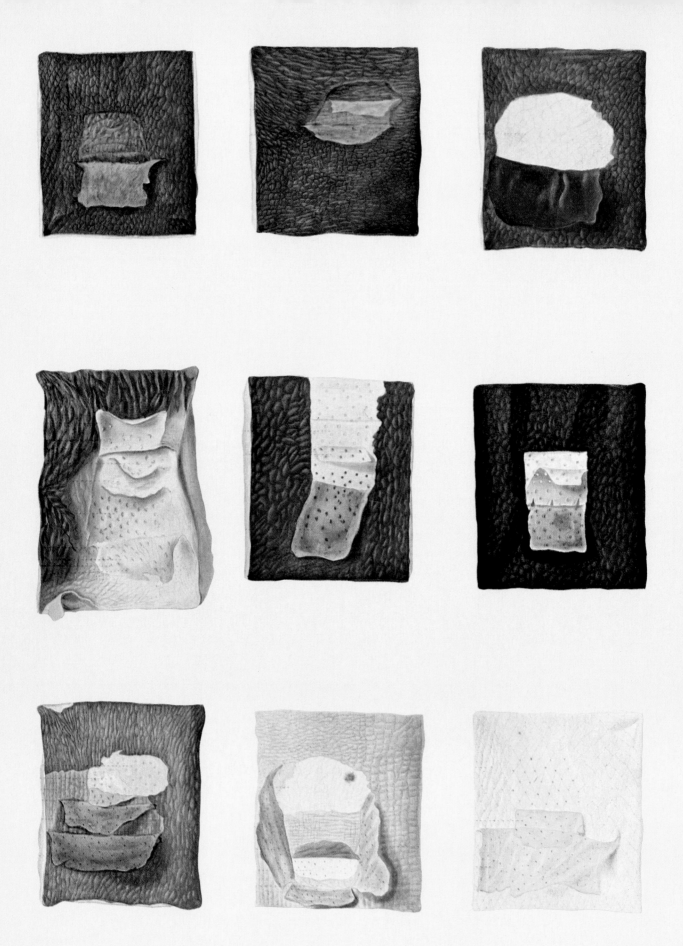

Pigment variation from Anatomie Générale de la Peau et des Membranes Muqueuses, *by Pierre Flourens, 1845.*

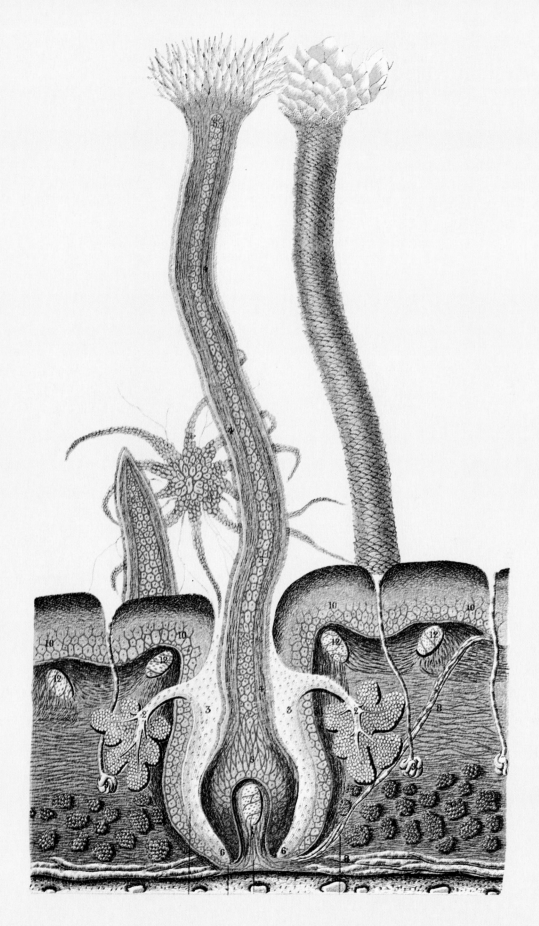

Anatomy of the hair from De L'Epiderme et de ses Variétés, *by H.M. du Malmont, 1866.*

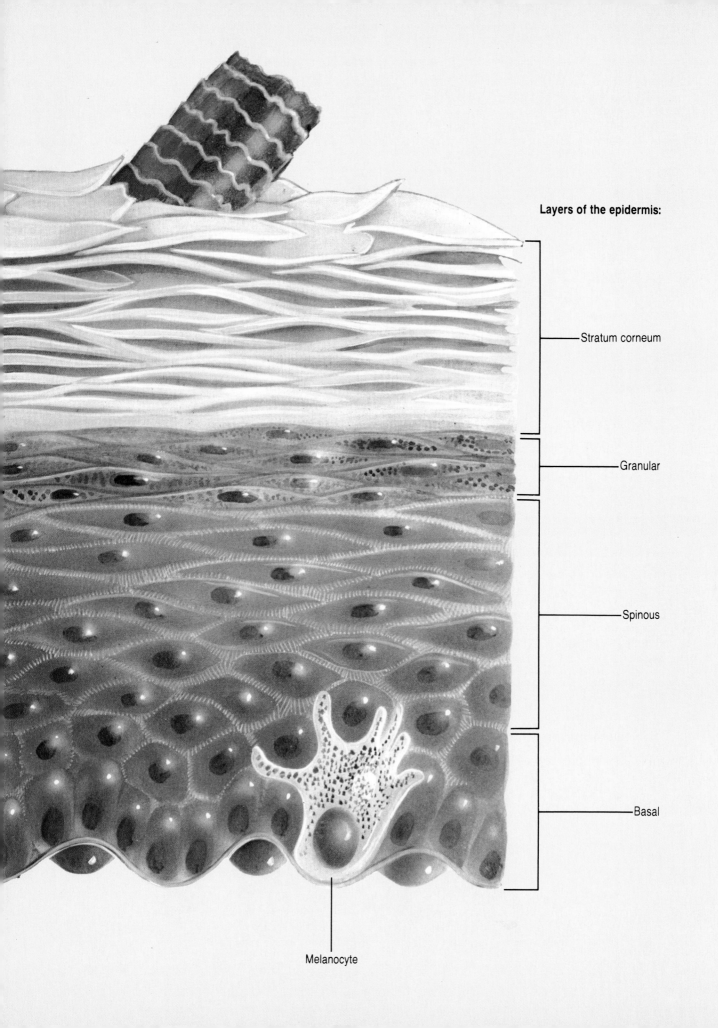

Layers of the epidermis:

Stratum corneum

Granular

Spinous

Basal

Melanocyte

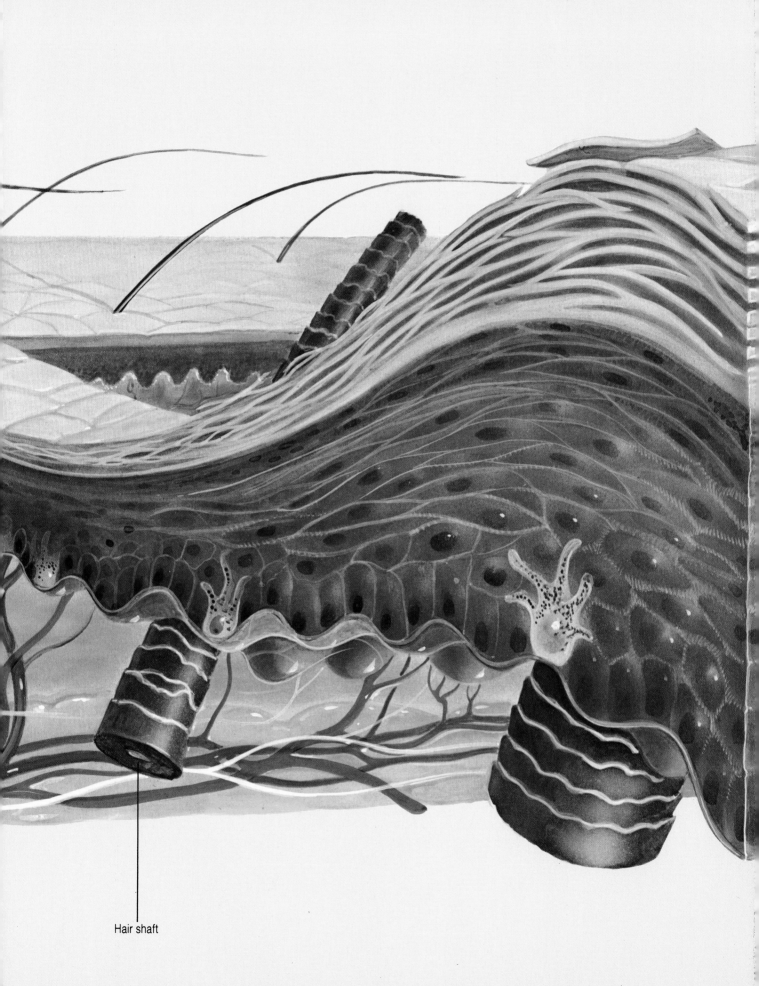

Hair shaft

Henry Faulds

Nature's Witness

Walking along the cliffs of Tokyo Bay one day in the late 1870s, Henry Faulds chanced upon a curious sight. Among the scattered fragments of prehistoric pottery there were pieces that bore the ancient potters' fingerprints, pressed into the clay when still soft. The impressions made thousands of years earlier led Faulds on a quest to discover how fingerprints varied among individuals, families, races and even different species.

A Scottish physician, Faulds served in India and in Japan as a medical missionary. Arriving in Tokyo in 1874, he stayed eleven years and in that time established a hospital, a medical school and a medical journal. He also cultivated his hobby of studying fingerprints. His position and the assistance of Japanese medical students afforded him a rich opportunity to collect and compare prints. In time, he began to correspond with scientists in England, including Charles Darwin, the distinguished naturalist. Faulds surmised that no two people had identical fingerprints. By offering his help to police, he helped to prove one suspected criminal's guilt and another's innocence by inspecting the fingerprints left at the scenes of the crimes.

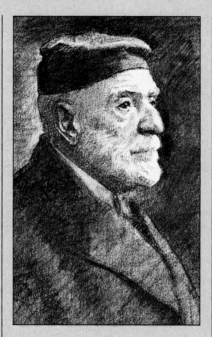

Convinced of the practical importance of fingerprinting, Faulds sent a letter in 1880 to the English science magazine, *Nature*. It summarized his work in Japan and his thoughts about the usefulness of fingerprinting. Faulds wrote that police departments should have in their files not only photographic records but also a "nature-copy of the forever-unchanging finger-furrows of important criminals." He also described how fingerprints helped convict one suspect and absolve another. His letter was the first published reference to fingerprints and their use in identifying criminals.

Faulds' letter to *Nature* brought an immediate response from Sir William J. Herschel, who claimed to have been using fingerprints as a means of identification for twenty years. As the administrator of the Hooghly district in Bengal, India, Herschel routinely required fingerprints from pensioners to make sure that no one was paid twice. For years, Faulds and Herschel carried on a lively exchange in the pages of *Nature* over claims of who originated the idea of fingerprint identification. Faulds, in the meantime, wrote a number of books on fingerprints and for a while published a bimonthly journal on fingerprints, *Dactylography*.

Shortly after returning to Great Britain from Japan in 1886, Faulds suggested that the English police establish a fingerprint bureau at Scotland Yard. He offered to help set up the office at no pay. His plan was considered but was ultimately rejected on the grounds that fingerprinting was too complex for routine criminal investigations. Scotland Yard's deductions proved false in this case, however. Faulds was vindicated within two decades as fingerprints became the preferred means of identification by police in Europe, England and the United States.

prints leading from the scene of the murder to the boy's bedroom belonged to his stepmother.

Modern fingerprinting stems from the work of several seventeenth-century European scientists, among them Malpighi, who identified the dermal papillae and the sweat pores of the skin ridges. Malpighi first associated the dermal papillae with touch, finding them larger and more numerous "particularly in places endowed with a more exquisite sense of touch." In 1684, English botanist Nehemiah Grew first described ridge patterns as "very regularly disposed into Spherical Triangles and Ellipticks" in a report to the Royal Society. Sweat pores along the ridges could be seen with the naked eye. But with a magnifying glass, he wrote, "every Pore looks like a little Fountain, and the sweat may be seen to stand therein, as clear as rock water, and as often as it is wiped off, to spring up within them again."

Nearly a century and a half later, Bohemian physician Johannes Evangelist Purkinje described nine distinct fingerprint patterns that roughly match the categories of modern identification systems. In 1880, Henry Faulds, a Scottish physician, suggested that fingerprints be used to help capture criminals. English astronomer and inventor Sir Francis Galton, turning his eye to the study of fingerprints in the 1880s, formulated a detailed classification system that would influence many scientists and law-enforcement investigators around the world. In a textbook published in 1892, Galton advised that fingerprints were "an incomparably surer criterion of identity than any other bodily feature."

Mark Twain's fascination for Galton's book prompted him to write *The Tragedy of Pudd'nhead Wilson*, a novel about a small-town Mississippi murder and the lawyer who solves it by finding fingerprints on the murder weapon. Convincing the jury, "These marks are his signature, his physiological autograph, so to speak . . . that cannot . . . become illegible by the wear and mutations of time," Pudd'nhead clears the two accused men, identifies the real murderer and unravels a tangled plot of baby switching and mixed identities.

By the time Twain's book was published in 1894, the use of fingerprints had already made

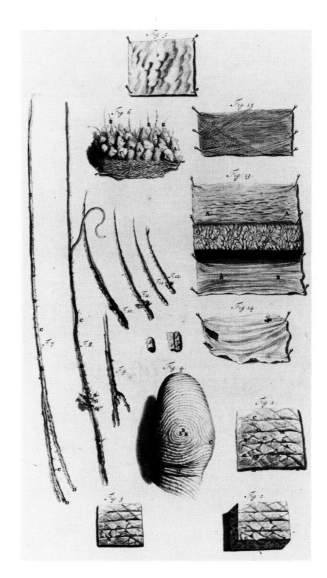

Along with his contemporaries Marcello Malpighi and Nehemiah Grew, seventeenth-century Dutch anatomist Govard Bidloo also traced the variety of texture that is skin's. These illustrations from Bidloo's Anatomia Humani Corporis, *printed in 1685, show several swatches of skin, including a whorled thumb pattern. Failing to appreciate the distinctive design of each fingertip, Bidloo overlooked their use as means of identification.*

the transition from fiction to everyday practice. Two doctors, both inspired by Galton's writings, developed identification systems. Juan Vucetich devised a method of identification adopted in 1891 by the police of La Plata, Argentina — the first system to be officially endorsed. Vucetich's system is still used in Argentina and several other South American countries. Within two years, Sir Edward Henry, the British inspector assigned to Bengal, India, introduced a similar system for identification. Soon adopted in England, the Henry system established the foundation for classification methods used in most English-speaking countries today.

Advocates of fingerprinting for identification encountered resistance from many European police departments because another method of identification had already gained wide acceptance. During the 1880s and 1890s, French police inspector Alphonse Bertillon had developed a method of recording various body measurements to identify arrested criminals. No two people were thought to have the same measurements. Anthropometry, or bertillonage, as the system was called, aided in the solution of a number of important crimes. But bertillonage began to lose ground to fingerprinting around the turn of the century because of the greater reliability and ease in recording fingerprints. Ironically, Bertillon was the first to solve a crime on the basis of fingerprints alone when he cracked a burglary case in Paris in 1902.

Advances in the detection and comparison of prints have improved criminal investigation greatly since the turn of the century. Some criminals have tried to remove the skin ridges on their fingertips with acid. In the 1930s, the infamous John Dillinger underwent unsuccessful operations to remove his fingerprints. Unless the dermal skin layer is severely damaged, however, the ridges will reappear in their original pattern.

When investigating crimes, early detectives relied on prints left by blood, soot or some other highly visible substance. Today, a number of techniques enable investigators to examine and record fingerprints not easily seen by the naked eye. A latent print remains when the sweat pores along the skin ridges of the fingertip leave an outline. Since the pores ooze tiny beads of sweat continuously, it is impossible not to leave a print on most surfaces. But because 99 percent of sweat is water, most of the print evaporates, leaving behind scant traces of salt, amino acids and fat. Powders and chemicals, such as iodine and silver nitrate, are commonly applied to illuminate fingerprints. More recently, laser beams have proved successful in experimental detection on unusual surfaces, including skin tissue itself. At the Federal Bureau of Investigation, computer technology aids the comparison of fingerprints, a recent innovation that should improve the ability to sort more than 175 million fingerprints.

Fingerprints have yielded a bounty of useful information in the years since Nehemiah Grew first studied them. Shortly before he applied scientific scrutiny to the lines of the finger ridges, an amateur Dutch scientist made a discovery that would open a whole new world to inquiry. In 1676, Anton van Leeuwenhoek described the bacteria he saw through one of his microscopes. Since his first glimpse, undreamed of populations of plant and animal life have been uncovered in the environment and on man himself.

Skin's Residents

Human skin appears lifeless to the naked eye much as the Earth appears uniformly still and lifeless from a thousand miles away. But the number of living organisms on a person's skin roughly equals the number of people on the planet. Like Earth, skin harbors life. The various inhabitants live in an interdependent network of delicately balanced communities. Could they speak, they might describe their surroundings much as the Lilliputian who told Gulliver he "could discover great Holes in my skin; that the Stumps of my Beard were ten Times stronger than the Bristles of a Boar; and my Complexion made up of several Colors altogether disagreeable." Far from unwelcome visitors to be washed off in a shower, the fauna and flora of the skin are permanent residents. Harmful organisms attract the most attention, but the overwhelming majority of the inhabitants are harmless. The use of antibiotics to kill harmful organisms may severely disrupt the balance of life on the skin.

52

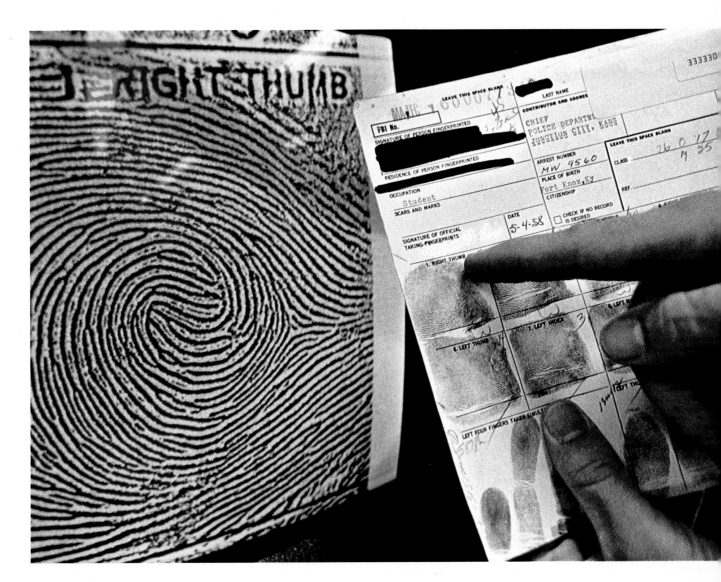

Quickening the hand and sharpening the eye of technicians working at the Federal Bureau of Investigation, computers hasten classification and identification of fingerprints. A scanner flashes a thumb print onto a monitor, highlighting the features that distinguish it from every other thumb in the world. The automated equipment can scan a fingerprint in half a second and match it to one of the more than 175 million prints on file in four seconds.

Trying Job's faith in vain, Satan smites him with boils in William Blake's nineteenth-century rendering of the biblical passage. Boils are no less infernal for being caused by a bacterium.

Yawning cavernously, the mouth of a single sweat gland, right, harbors bacteria clinging to its walls like bats. Seemingly baleful yet surely benign, these bacteria mix with sweat to produce body odor.

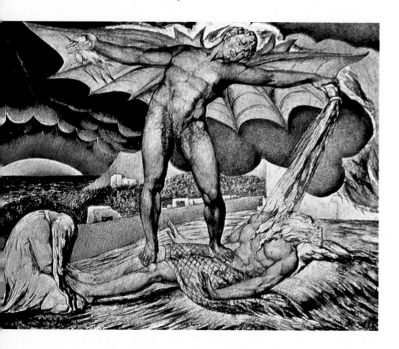

The skin varies immensely from one region of the body to another. Different populations of bacteria and yeasts have adapted to specific environments. The dry expanse of the forearm, the dense tangle of the scalp and the oily surface of the nose all harbor particular organisms.

One of the largest residents of the skin lives in the hair follicles of the eyelashes, nose, chin and scalp of most adults. A narrow, wormlike mite, *Demodex folliculorum* lives most of its life in the hair follicle and lays its eggs in the sebaceous glands that supply the follicle with sebum. The young molt twice in the follicle, then journey across the skin at night in search of another follicle to inhabit. Although the *Demodex* mite was identified in 1842, no one has discovered what it eats or what role it plays in the balance of the skin's life. Others, such as the red chigger and the scabies mite, sometimes live on skin, but only *Demodex* has made its home there.

The chigger and scabies mites are parasites. The female scabies mite burrows just beneath the skin's surface in the corneal layer, usually on the hands and wrists, inside the elbows and around the genitals. In tunnels about an inch long, it lays eggs which hatch in three or four days. After several weeks, the infected person develops an itchy allergic reaction. Scabies are passed from person to person by close physical contact. The application of a benzyl benzoate solution to the skin eliminates the mites. The chigger finds its way to man via grass and bushes. Chiggers feed on blood and leave small red swellings, usually on the legs. A sulfur ointment containing phenol gets rid of them.

Bacteria make up the largest community on the skin. Simple, one-celled organisms, most bacteria have no power of locomotion and rely on their immediate surroundings for nourishment. By breaking down dead matter into its constituent parts, bacteria provide an important link in the world's food chains. Although the functions of bacteria on the skin are not completely understood, some residents benefit their host. Others are generally harmless. *Corynebacterium acnes* thrives in the depths of the hair follicle where oxygen is scarce. This bacterium also contributes to acne. Another species, *Staphylococcus aureus*, is dangerous. If staph bacteria enter the blood stream, they can cause a fatal infection. They reproduce rapidly in the blood and have the ability to build up resistance to antibiotics, which makes the infection more difficult to treat.

People acquire bacteria on the skin at birth. In natural deliveries, babies pick up bacteria when passing through the mother's vagina. A baby delivered by Caesarean will also pick up bacteria in the air and from contact with people. In the days following birth, the bacteria population grows rapidly. Within a day, bacteria in the armpit will number about 6,000 per square centimeter. In another four days, their number reaches 24,000 and, by the ninth day, the population levels off at around 81,000. Bacteria spread from person to person both by contact and by constant shedding of skin cells, at the rate of more than a million every hour.

Bacteria become established on a baby's skin on a first-come, first-served basis, depending on what types of bacteria happen to be in the delivery room and around the hospital. Once such populations become established on the skin, they fill the niches in the skin's environment that harmful bacteria could otherwise occupy. The resident bacteria will fight off intruding competi-

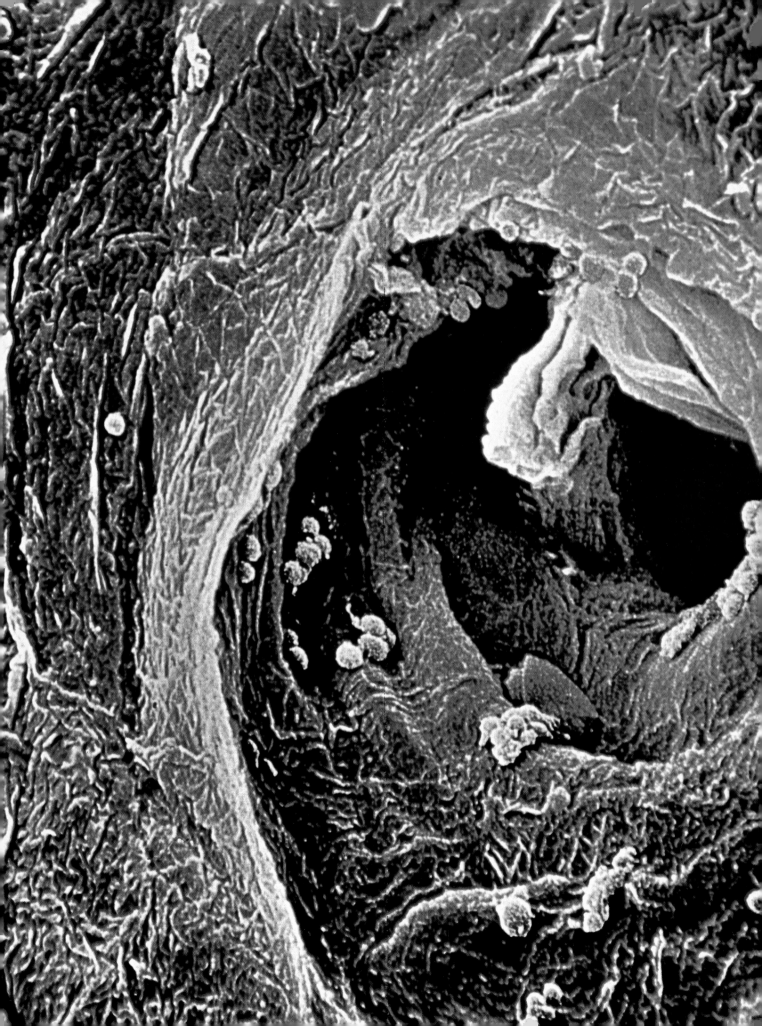

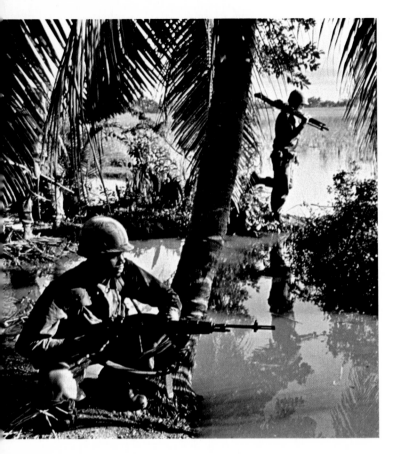

infection arising from trekking through rice paddies and swamps. Various skin diseases ranked high among the hazards of the Vietnam War. Another bacterial infection caused by saturation of the skin occurs in less hazardous surroundings. The bacterium *Pseudomonas* afflicts many devotees of the hot tub with a rash known as hot tub itch.

Although they rely on the skin's environment for survival, not all of the skin's resident bacteria are freeloaders. Some bacteria thrive in flesh wounds, protecting the body by producing an antibiotic that wards off harmful bacteria. The natural populations of the skin may serve the health of their human hosts in many ways that are yet unknown.

Viruses, the smallest life forms inhabiting the skin, can be seen only with the aid of electron microscopes. Since the outer layer of skin has no living cells, a virus must live in the deeper layers. Unable to reproduce outside a host cell, the virus multiplies by tricking living cells into reproducing its own genetic material. When the host cell has produced more viruses than the cell can accommodate, the cell breaks open and the viruses move on to reproduce in other cells.

Named after the Latin for "slime" or "poison," viruses can cause serious illnesses. Herpes viruses are responsible for cold sores, chicken pox, infectious mononucleosis and shingles. Entering the skin through a cut or through the soft tissues of the mouth or genitals, the viruses multiply and form lesions. Of the seventy varieties of herpes viruses, herpes simplex is one of the most common. It appears in two forms. Herpes simplex I resides in the head causing cold sores and encephalitis, a dangerous brain infection. Herpes simplex II lives below the waist and causes genital herpes. However, Type I can infect the genital region and Type II can infect the head.

The incidence of genital herpes has risen to alarming proportions in recent years. Health professionals estimate that between five and twenty million Americans carry the virus. It is usually transmitted by sexual contact. Approximately three weeks after infection, the blisters that accompany genital herpes disappear. But the virus remains dormant in nerve centers in the lower back and returns to reinfect the skin periodically.

tors. Because there are so many types of bacteria and because each person develops a bacterial profile largely by chance, one professor has proposed that bacteriological techniques be added to criminal investigations.

In addition to the skirmishing lines of resident bacteria, the skin relies on several other defensive stratagems to ward off harmful microorganisms. Daily skin loss prevents many would-be colonists from gaining a foothold on the skin. The skin also presents an acidic mantle that deters some types of bacteria. When the skin's bacteria break down sebum, fatty acids that increase the skin's acidity are produced.

Bacteria thrive in moist areas, so the dryness of the skin probably accounts for most of its resistance to bacterial infections. When skin becomes too moist, its resistance decreases and bacteria break through normal defenses. American soldiers in Vietnam suffered from "paddy foot," an

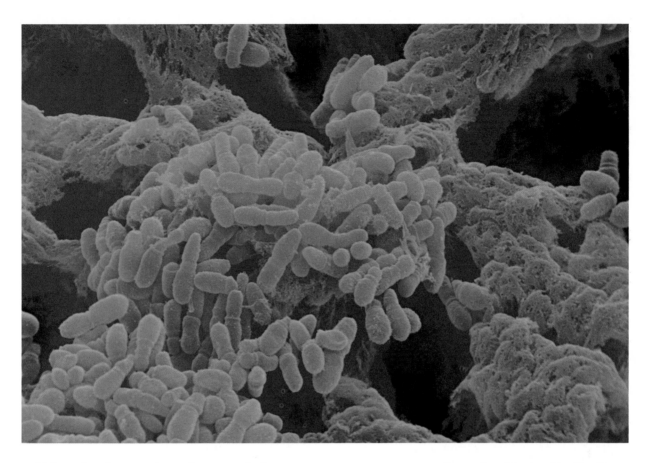

Although advances have been made in treatment, no cure for herpes exists. The study and treatment of the virus is hampered by its hibernation in nerve cells. Ointment containing the drug acyclovir has shown promising results. The drug prevents infected cells from producing herpes virus DNA, the genetic material necessary for its reproduction.

Plant life also flourishes on the skin in the form of fungus. Varieties of yeasts and dermatophytes cause common ailments. Yeasts grow in warm, moist areas, feeding on glucose, a sugar found in the body. Yeast infections sometimes arise when antibiotics upset the life balance on the skin. When the bacteria competing with yeasts for food are killed by the antibiotic, yeast populations multiply rapidly, overstepping their ecological niche. On the greasy surfaces of the nose, scalp and ears, the yeast *Pityrosporum ovale* can grow in numbers up to a half-million per

Consuming fats stored in the skin, Pityrosporum ovale, a yeast, thrives on the oily surfaces of the nose, scalp and ears. Unlike other yeasts that can spawn irritating infections, it is believed harmless.

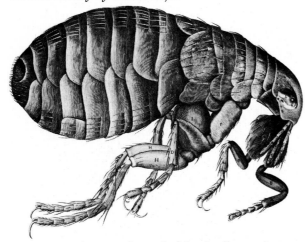

square centimeter. It probably feeds on fats in the skin and is believed to be harmless. Fungi also need moisture and dampness to survive. Suitable environments for their growth are the feet, where they cause athlete's foot, and in the groin, where they cause itching in men. Such infections produce scaly skin.

Ringworm, a fungal infection that has nothing to do with worms, derives its name from the appearance of circular patches of red, scaly skin. Ringworm begins as a small, infected patch that spreads out. Although the lesion starts to heal at the center, the healing cannot catch up with the spreading fungus, so a patch of healthy skin appears at the center of the red ring. Ringworm can infect the scalp, beard, body and nails. Perhaps because their immune systems are not fully developed, children are more frequently its victims than adults. House pets and people spread the infection. It is a stubborn ailment that requires two or three weeks of treatment to eliminate. Ointments containing clotrimazole or miconazole, both potent antifungal agents, can curb the infection. If local treatment is ineffective, the antibiotic griseofulvin can be taken orally.

Much larger and plainly visible, fleas also visit the body, but less commonly now than in the past. A modern romantic is unlikely to rhyme to his lover with John Donne, who wrote in the sixteenth century:

> Marke but this flea, and marke in this,
> How little that which thou deny'st me is;
> It suck'd me first, and now sucks thee,
> And in this flea, our two bloods mingled bee.

Fleas like those who shared Donne's intimacies have suffered a decline in population thanks to gradual improvements in hygiene. Other fleas fare well in clean, dry houses. Opportunists arriving via cats and dogs, the domestic variety also bite people. Fleas feed on blood, injecting their saliva into the skin to stop the host's blood from clotting. The saliva causes swelling. Given a choice, fleas seem to prefer women to men. The preference may be related to the advantage that rabbit fleas gain from their female hosts. The female rabbit flea relies on the hormones in the blood of a pregnant rabbit to trigger its own ovulation. Reacting to another hormonal signal from the rabbit when it gives birth, the flea migrates to a newborn rabbit where it mates and lays eggs, ensuring survival for another generation.

Fleas Most Foul

Although fleas attached to tiny chariots and carriages once entertained throngs of people at flea circuses, they also played a more sinister role in human affairs. Thirty species of flea transmit bacteria that cause plague. The plague bacterium *Yersinia pestis* thrives in underground tunnels where large numbers of burrowing rodents live. When rat fleas become infected, they pass the disease to the rats which eventually die from plague. The fleas abandon the dying rats in search of a new source of food, and since rats often live near humans, the fleas find their way to man. Once in the flea, the bacteria reproduce rapidly in its gut, forming a block that prevents the flea from getting food into its body. In its vain, frenzied efforts to feed, the flea bites again and again. With each bite it regurgitates as many as 100,000 plague bacteria into the body of its host. At last the flea starves to death, but not before infecting its victim.

Unless the human immune system musters strong defenses, the bacteria multiply, often in the lymph glands of the armpit or the groin, to form a large and painful lump. The lump, which can become fist-sized, is called a bubo — hence the term bubonic plague. Plague afflicts the blood stream, causing blood to leak from capillaries. The Black Death earned its name from the dark color of blood seeping beneath the skin.

*"All diseases of Christians,"
St. Augustine preached, "are to be
ascribed to demons." The plague
demon in this German woodcut of
1540 cast Christendom under the
shadow of the Black Death.*

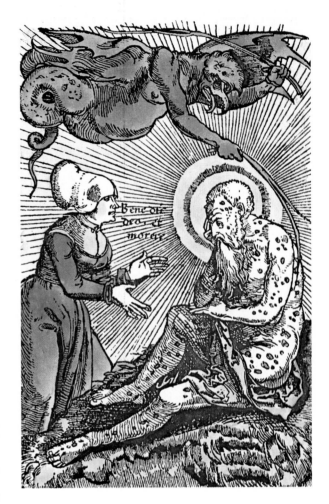

Compounded by pneumonia, plague takes its most virulent form, passing on droplets of moisture released by sneezing and coughing.

Throughout the ages, plague struck human populations repeatedly, often ravaging entire societies. Plague probably contributed to the fall of the Roman Empire. In the year 540, during the rule of the emperor Justinian I, plague spread from Egypt across the empire. In Byzantium, it killed as many as 10,000 a day. Historian Edward Gibbon concluded that 100 million Romans may have died as a result of the Justinian plague. He described the emperor's reign as "disgraced by a visible decrease of the human species."

Between the eleventh and seventeenth centuries, plague struck Europe many times. An outbreak beginning in 1346, which occasioned the phrase "the Black Death," killed a quarter of the population of Europe. A million Egyptians were carried off by the disease in 1603, and 300,000 Neapolitans succumbed in 1656. The plague remained a continual threat in Europe well into the eighteenth century, when advances in medicine and sanitation restricted its toll.

When plague at Marseilles threatened to spread from France to England in 1721, English novelist Daniel Defoe wrote *A Journal of the Plague Year,* an account of the great plague that had ravaged London in 1665 to alert his readers to its danger. Drawing upon vivid contemporary accounts, Defoe described the solemn terror of mass burials, carts for the dead heaped with victims and the call at the homes of the stricken: "Bring out your dead." Explaining the outbreak, Defoe declared, "Nothing but the immediate finger of God, nothing but omnipotent power, could have done it." He thought the affliction could be detected by breathing on a glass "where, the breath condensing, there might living creatures be seen by a microscope, of strange, monstrous, and frightful shapes, such as dragons, snakes, serpents, and devils, horrible to behold."

Almost an apocalyptic menace, it earned a place in folklore and myth. A common malediction of Shakespearean times, "May the plague take you," was more than an idle threat. The children's rhyme, "Ring around the rosy," may take its origins from sights made familiar by the

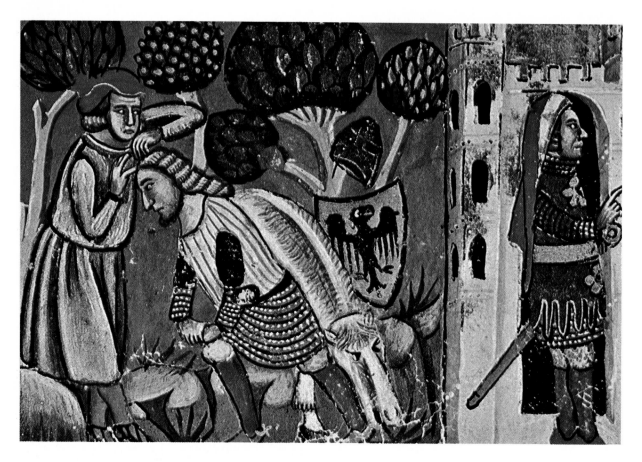

plague. "Rosy" may refer to the rash that broke out on the faces of plague victims, and a "pocketful of posies" may signify the herbs and spices carried as a folk remedy and as perfume. The concluding line, "all fall down," might then be nothing more than an enactment of the inevitable fate of those stricken with the plague.

The discovery of the plague's cause and the identification of its carriers did not happen until the end of the nineteenth century. Plague persists in the twentieth century, but the extermination of rats and the development of antibiotics have helped reduce its fatal consequences.

Like the flea, the body louse is easily seen by the naked eye. And, like certain species of flea, body lice spread disease. Typhus is caused by *Rickettsia prowazeki,* a microorganism that infects and kills lice. Although lice feed on human blood by piercing the skin, the *Rickettsiae*-laden excrement of the body louse usually accounts for the spread of typhus. Because body lice lay their eggs in the lining of clothing, typhus was once a common disease among soldiers at war who had little chance to wash or change clothes. Between 1917 and 1923, typhus killed three million people in Russia. The insecticide DDT helped to curb typhus during World War II. Today, a vaccine guards against the spread of typhus, and antibiotics effectively treat the disease.

Two other kinds of lice that live on the body have increased their numbers greatly in recent years. The crab louse and the head louse currently make their home on millions of people and appear to be spreading rapidly. The crab louse lives most frequently in the pubic hair and occasionally in the hair of the armpits, beard and eyebrows. This louse is almost always transmitted during sexual intercourse. The head louse resides on a large proportion of schoolchildren in the United States and elsewhere. The close physical

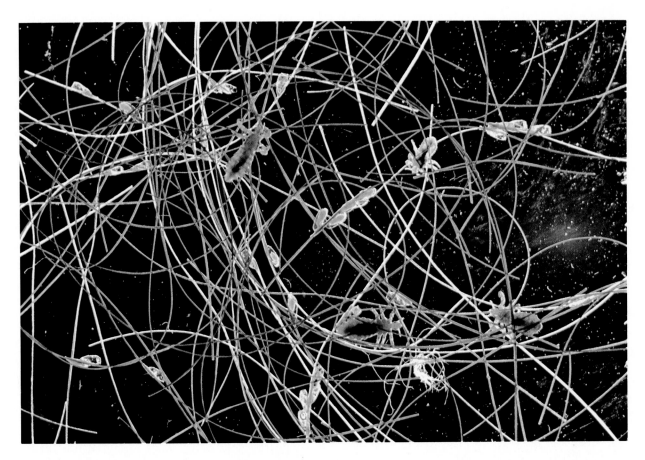

contact among children may explain the spread. The head louse attaches its eggs, or nits, to hairs near the scalp. The tedious business of searching for the eggs and picking them out of the hair demonstrates the literal meaning of the term "nit picking." The attraction hair holds for the louse once supplied the means of choosing political leadership in medieval Hurdenburg, Sweden. Candidates for mayor gathered around a table, with their beards touching the tabletop. The new mayor was considered chosen when a louse dropped in the middle of the table crawled to the beard of its choice.

Swarming with settlers and circled by raiders, the skin is a bustling frontier, alive with the commerce between man's body and his world. Skin constantly renews itself, yet remains a firm and fixed boundary. Its tapestry distinguishes man from his surroundings as surely as the patterns of its weave distinguish men from one another.

Stubborn squatters on the scalp, lice shelter and reproduce amid slender strands of hair. From painstaking efforts to evict them and their off-spring, nits — one by one — comes the expression "nit picking."

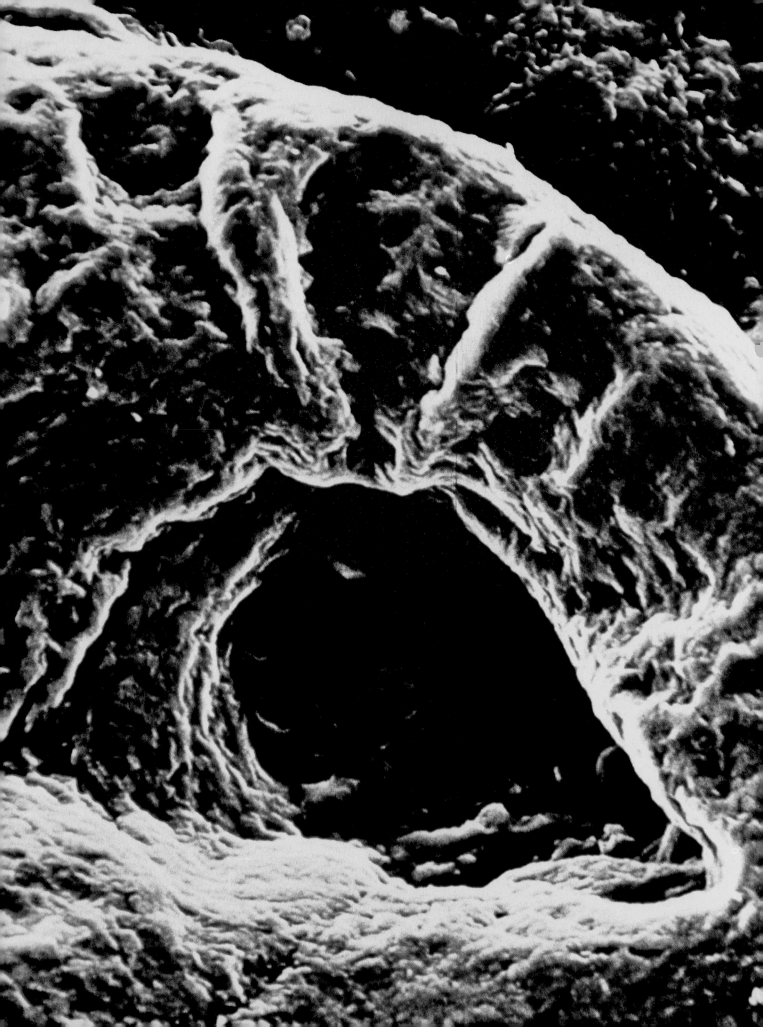

Chapter 3

Barrier to the World

Anything that penetrates the body must first confront the skin. Skin is a living boundary that separates the inside of the body from the world. Constantly in contact with the environment, it is tough enough to resist countless chemical and environmental assaults, yet soft and sensitive enough to respond to the gentlest touch. A versatile organ, skin provides first-line defense against invading organisms and other foreign substances, all the while regulating movement of substances from the interior to the exterior. Our bodies are made mostly of water — as much as 75 percent at birth and somewhat less later in life. Skin protects the body from its considerably drier surroundings.

The barrier, however, is selectively penetrable. Skin secretes fluids that lubricate it, barricade toxic substances and maintain a stable internal environment. It absorbs other substances, particularly those soluble in oils. This absorptive function has proved effective in administering certain medications. Through the skin, drugs enter the underlying circulatory system in steady doses. Small adhesive patches, worn behind the ears and replaced daily, deliver a motion-sickness remedy. Others, applied to the chest, administer medicine to relieve the pain of angina pectoris, caused by an insufficient supply of blood to the heart. These, too, are replaced every day.

Skin is also a prominent part of the body's temperature-regulating system. The job is a constant one, requiring small adjustments to ensure that internal temperature, the body's core temperature, does not stray from the narrow range at which the organs function most efficiently. This temperature, differing slightly from person to person, averages 98.6° F. Called the set point, it is analogous to a setting on a thermostat. The system is so delicately balanced that if the core temperature varies one-and-a-half degrees, the body's metabolism is altered by about 20 percent.

Magnified 1,500 times, a pore in human skin becomes a portal between inner and outer worlds. The skin is the body's boundary, an invaluable barrier between man and the environment. Skin is also a sensitive regulatory organ. Through millions of pores like this one, it protects the body from extremes of heat and exertion.

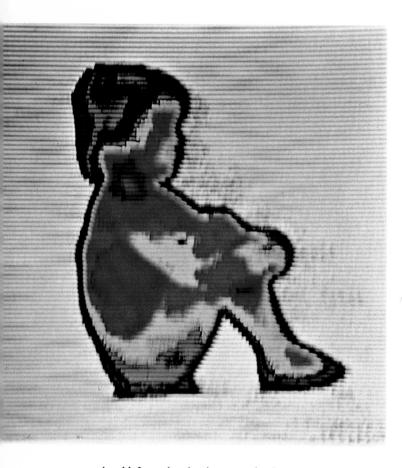

A cold floor absorbs the warmth of the child seated upon it. Vibrant red reflects the warmest portions of the body, while blue and green indicate the coolest — areas releasing more heat to the surroundings.

When body temperature shifts slightly from the set point, the heating or cooling mechanism quickly restores the proper temperature. The skin regulates body temperature largely by controlling the amount of heat lost. To do so, it works in concert with the hypothalamus, a cluster of nerve cells at the center of the brain. Specialized regions of the hypothalamus contain heat-sensitive and cold-sensitive cells that respond to changes in blood temperature by increasing the number of nerve impulses they transmit. On command, the skin hastens to make the appropriate adjustments in its domain.

Even in stable surroundings, this temperature-regulating system functions all the time, for although the body constantly produces heat, it also constantly loses heat. In a moderate room temperature, the body loses most heat through what scientists call radiation — rays of heat that emanate in all directions. Other objects in the room constantly radiate heat back to the body, but a body warmer than its surroundings always loses more heat than it gains.

When touching something, the body conducts heat to the object's surface. The warmth of a chair someone is sitting in represents heat loss through conduction. But only a small amount of heat is lost in this way. Within a few minutes, the temperature of the chair seat will match the body's surface temperature. At that point, the chair seat becomes an insulator, preventing much additional heat loss. Even when the body is not touching something else, it can still lose heat through conduction because it is always in contact with air molecules. As with the chair, once the temperature of the surrounding air is equal to the body's, heat loss from body to air will cease.

In a draft of cool air, the body also loses heat continuously. The heat, carried away by the air currents, is lost by convection. Because air rises as it gets warmer, convection always occurs around the body even though there are no noticeable currents. Convection accounts for about 12 percent of heat loss from a person seated in a still room. Drafts increase heat loss by replacing surrounding air more rapidly.

When submerged in water, the body loses heat through conduction and convection much more

Exposed to the cold, skin conserves body heat, left. Tiny muscles called arrector pili pull hairs erect to trap a layer of insulating air next to the skin. Junctions between tiny veins and arteries, arteriovenous anasto- *moses, constrict to reduce the flow of blood to the skin's cool surface. Hot weather or strenuous exercise prompts a different process, right. Sweat glands pour water onto the skin so that evaporation can cool the* *body. Anastomoses open wide to bring more blood to the skin, where body warmth can be shed into the surrounding air. The arrector pili then relax, allowing damp hair to lie close to the skin.*

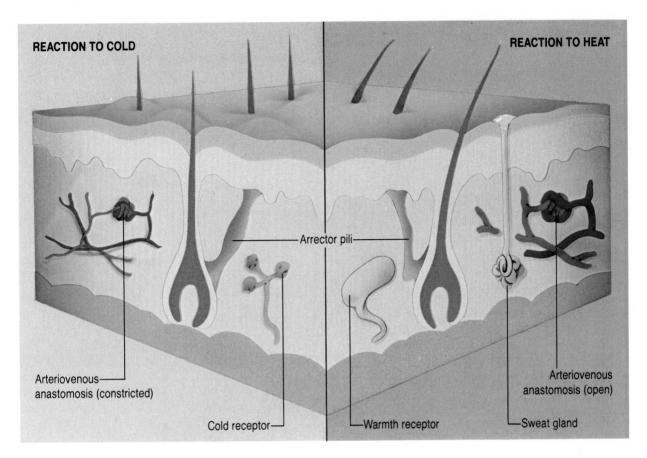

REACTION TO COLD **REACTION TO HEAT**

Arrector pili

Arteriovenous anastomosis (constricted)

Cold receptor

Warmth receptor

Arteriovenous anastomosis (open)

Sweat gland

quickly because water is a much better conductor of heat. Even when water and air are the same temperature, the body loses much more heat in water. But the ratios even up somewhat when both air and water are extremely cold. Then, both are almost equally capable of drawing heat away from the body.

Evaporation of insensible perspiration is another means by which heat is continuously lost. This differs from sweating in that it is usually not noticeable. The body loses about twenty to thirty grams of water — about an ounce — in an hour. Two-thirds of the lost fluid comes from interstitial fluid in the dermis, fluid between cells in the deepest layer of skin. The rest of the fluid evaporates through the respiratory passages. Dogs pant to increase heat loss in this way.

When the core temperature drops, alarms sound throughout the body. Because the hypothalamus has relatively few cold-sensitive nerve cells, the decreased action of its heat-sensitive neurons helps indicate the need to conserve heat. These nerve cells usually become inactive by the time body temperature has dropped a few tenths of a degree, however. There are cold sensors in other areas of the central nervous system, but most cold detection occurs on the body's periphery, which contains abundant specialized nerve endings called thermoreceptors. The skin has far more cold receptors than warmth receptors. The number of cold receptors also varies from one region of the body to the next. The skin on the lips contains about twenty times more cold receptors than the skin on the chest and legs.

Cold receptors send their signals up the spinal cord to the hypothalamus, which sends impulses to structures in skin called arteriovenous anastomoses, specialized connections between veins and arteries that intermittently substitute for capillaries throughout the circulatory system and

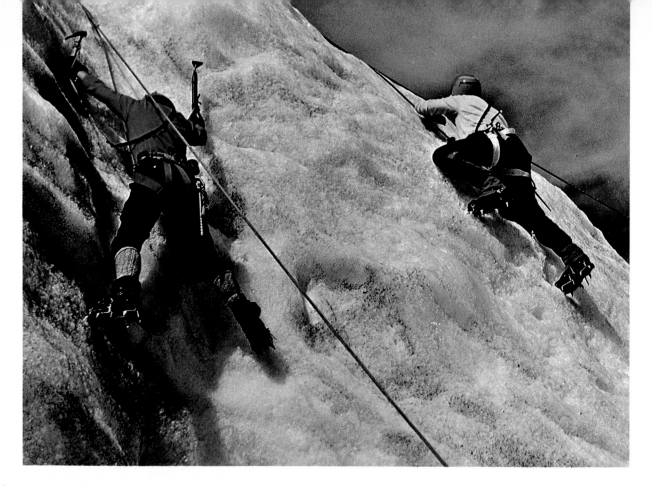

reroute blood flow. They are particularly abundant in the hands and feet, eyelids, nose and lips. The middle portion of an anastomosis is a thick, muscular wall that contracts, restricting blood flow to the extremities and thus reducing heat loss. This is why our lips and fingernails take on a slightly blue cast when we are cold — lending truth to the saying "cold hands, warm heart."

With restricted blood flow, "goose bumps," tiny lumps caused by erection of the hair shafts, appear on the skin. This action, piloerection, is largely useless in man. In animals, it makes fur stand on end and helps create an extra layer of warmth by trapping more air next to the body.

The body also reacts to cooling by increasing its metabolic activity. In particular, its skeletal muscles, the large voluntary muscles, will increase their action. As the body gets colder, muscle tension builds, gradually leading to the tremors known as shivering. The synchronized muscular contractions occur at rates of ten to twenty per second, generating heat to warm the internal organs. Voluntary muscle movement such as stomping the feet and shaking the hands works toward the same end. Muscular contraction generates most of the body's heat. Prior to every contraction, a burst of chemical energy is released. Normally, most of the energy fuels the contraction, while the unused amount is released as heat. Shivering can actually warm the body more efficiently than voluntary contractions because it uses a smaller amount of chemical energy to fuel the work and, therefore, releases more heat. Strong shivering, which can cause heat production eight times higher than that of a person slowly moving about in a moderate room temperature, offers only limited protection. It warms the body only for the length of time it compensates for heat lost. If the environment draws more heat away than the body produces, body temperature will continue to fall.

When the body cannot completely offset heat loss, hypothermia, the drop in internal body temperature to 95° F or below, can occur. Such heat loss can be extremely dangerous. A skater who falls through the ice of a frozen pond can survive for twenty to thirty minutes. As body temperature falls, the central nervous system begins to work less efficiently. By the time core temperature has reached 91.4°, a person loses consciousness and the temperature-regulating mechanism slows down. As body temperature approaches 86°, the mechanism ceases functioning. Blood vessels become completely constricted. At a

This sheer cliff of ice threatens life and limb in more ways than one. When too long in contact with the freezing surface, climbers risk frostbite. Such exposure can claim body tissue, usually hands and feet.

Sweat looms large in importance as a cooling mechanism, but only when it is allowed to evaporate from the skin. These sweat droplets on the surface of the thumb are magnified 900 times.

slightly lower temperature, nerve transmission becomes so impaired that heartbeat is affected, and death follows rapidly.

If detected soon enough, hypothermia can be treated successfully. In a severe case, doctors may circulate the patient's blood through a hemodialysis machine, the same apparatus used to filter the blood of people whose kidneys malfunction. The hemodialyzer warms the blood and pumps it back into the body. By surrounding the body in ice or packing it in chilled blankets, doctors occasionally induce hypothermia before heart surgery to lower the patient's oxygen need and to enable surgeons to stop the heart for a longer time than is otherwise possible.

"The Edge of Agony"

In frostbite, tissue becomes so chilled that it freezes. Earlobes, fingers and toes are especially vulnerable. Barry Bishop was one of the first Americans to reach the summit of Mount Everest in 1963. Recording the descent, he noted, "My feet, warm and comfortable throughout the entire climb, now begin to freeze. I stamp ponderously in the snow. No help. The pain in my toes sharpens. Then, as it skirts the edge of agony, it dies in a merciful numbness." Bishop recognized the signs of frostbite. Pain returns to the region when it begins to thaw and that is when doctors can assess damage. Like burns, frostbite can be ranked by degrees of severity. In first-degree frostbite, the skin looks blistered and red. It feels hot and is accompanied by a stinging pain. This lasts for four to five days. Second-degree and third-degree frostbite, progressively more severe, affect deeper and deeper layers of skin. Pain and damage are also greater and more lasting. The most severe, fourth-degree, affects bone. Barry Bishop's battle with Mount Everest cost him several toes and fingertips.

Except for very mild cases, frostbite should be treated as soon as possible. Doctors often use a whirlpool bath heated to 107° F to restore the circulation. By simply wearing warm, waterproof, nonbinding clothing in cold weather, frostbite can be prevented.

The body reacts to excessive heat in an opposite fashion, taking measures to encourage heat

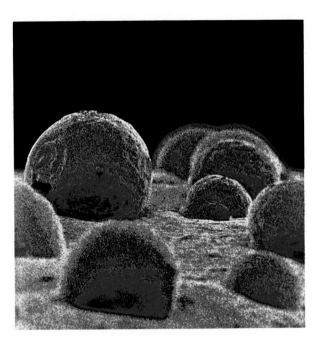

loss. Sweating begins and blood vessels throughout the skin dilate to allow more blood to reach the surface, just as water that cools a car's engine circulates through the radiator to become cooled. This allows the blood to dissipate more body heat and accounts for the flushed, rosy glow of the skin during exercise. This same mechanism causes blushing.

The layer of sweat that has built up on the skin's surface helps cool it by evaporating. Sweating is normally an effective cooling mechanism, particularly in a hot, dry environment. It can protect against degrees of heat that most people seldom experience. More than two centuries ago, British physician Sir Charles Blagden and several colleagues acted as test subjects in an experiment that would expose them to severe heat. As Blagden later recorded, he and his companions "all rejoiced at the opportunity of being convinced, by our own experience, of the wonderful power with which the animal body is endued, of resisting an heat vastly greater than its own temperature." Blagden entered a chamber heated to 260° F. Exposed to temperatures hot enough to fry a steak, he felt no great discomfort, even after fifteen minutes. "Upon touching my side it felt cold like a corpse," he wrote, "and yet the actual heat of my body, tried under my tongue, and by applying closely the thermometer to my skin, was 98°, about a degree higher than its ordinary temperature."

Sweat cools the body only when it is able to evaporate from the skin. In extremely humid weather, sweating can become dangerous by leading to dehydration without having any cooling effect. Dehydration can lead to a boost in body temperature, which, when twelve degrees above normal, offers little chance of survival.

Unrelenting Heat

A number of recent deaths, all with a curiously modern twist to them, speak of the dangers of submitting the body to unrelenting heat. In 1979, a man calling on friends in California was alarmed when they did not come to the door although he could hear the sound of water running in their backyard hot tub. He summoned the police, who found the couple, both dead, floating in their redwood tub. About a year later, a similar tragedy struck in a different setting. Two runners in a ten-mile marathon in Herndon, Virginia could not be accounted for at the race's end. Their bodies were later discovered. Both had collapsed within a mile of the finish line.

All had died of heat stroke, a dangerous illness brought on by extreme heat. Elevated body temperature is called hyperthermia. When it reaches 106° to 108°, the heart begins beating irregularly, the blood becomes depleted of oxygen and normal functioning of the liver ceases. Initially marked by dizziness and confusion, heat stroke can rapidly lead to unconsciousness and death if body temperature is not lowered. Humans rarely survive a body temperature of 110°. In each of the four deaths, the body's cooling mechanism was impaired. The California couple had set the temperature of the water in their hot tub at 114° — far above the recommended temperature of 102° to 104°. The water prevented their sweat from evaporating, causing their body temperature to climb without check.

The runners' environment was much the same. The marathon was run on a humid August day, with temperatures reaching into the nineties. The layout of the course offered little relief from the sun and the humidity prevented efficient evaporation of sweat. Distance running generates extreme body heat. Coupled with hot weather and humidity, the marathon was far more taxing than race officials had thought. The two men may have pushed their bodies too hard. Athletes can lose a half-gallon of water an hour when exercising on a hot, humid day, so doctors recommend drinking a cup or two of water every fifteen minutes to avoid dehydration and hyperthermia.

Hyperthermia is a sign of a struggle between the body and heat — one in which heat has the edge. There are times, however, when the body joins forces with heat, growing hotter not because heat is overpowering its thermoregulatory mechanism but because the mechanism has been altered to permit a higher than normal temperature. This is fever, the familiar symptom of many illnesses. The normal set point is raised, boosting the demand for heat. The body responds by increasing heat production and conservation.

Fever

Scientists' understanding of this mechanism is relatively recent. In 1948, researchers found that body temperature was reset not by an outside force but by a chemical produced in the body. The chemical later became known as endogenous pyrogen, a small protein produced by phagocytic white blood cells, cells that engulf and destroy invading bacteria and other substances. This self-protective action seems to encourage the production of endogenous pyrogen. Pyrogen travels through the blood to the brain, where it acts upon the thermoregulating region of the hypothalamus, apparently causing it to fix the set point at a higher temperature. Three groups of chemicals in the brain seem to be linked with resetting the set point. The most prominent are prostaglandins, a group of fatty acids. Their concentration in the brain increases when endogenous pyrogen is present. Aspirin reduces fever by preventing the formation of new prostaglandins. This helps the set point return to normal. The body then responds as it would to an overly warm environment. Blood moves to the surface of the skin to dissipate heat and we start to sweat. The fever is then said to break.

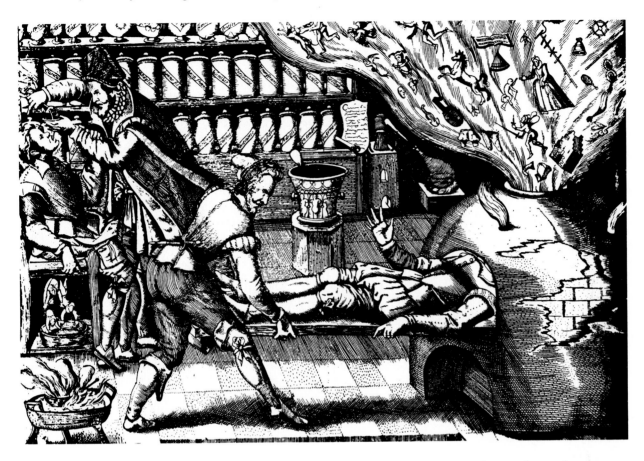

It is no wonder that with all the discomfort fever causes, we promptly act to treat it by taking aspirin. Constant companion to infection, fever has long been regarded as a conspirator in malaise and an evil in itself. Renowned nineteenth-century physician Sir William Osler placed fever among humanity's three great enemies, brother-in-arms to famine and war. Of them, he said, "by far the greatest, by far the most terrible, is fever."

Some scientists believe fever may be something of a benevolent force. Lizards injected with bacteria will bask in the sun until they raise their body temperatures to feverlike levels. If they are prevented from doing so, or if they are given aspirin, they will die of infection. Likewise, rabbits infected with bacteria are best able to recover when they run fevers about three degrees above their normal temperature. Their mortality rate increases when fevers run both above and below this moderate range.

There are indications that moderate fevers may be beneficial to humans, as well. Fever seems to reduce the level of iron in the blood and, by doing so, may help to reduce invading bacteria and fungi that need more iron to survive high temperatures. Both white blood cells and interferon, a virus-fighting protein in the body, seem to work more efficiently at higher temperatures. There is no evidence, however, that allowing a fever to progress without treatment improves a patient's recovery time or that reducing a fever prolongs an illness. High fever is certainly dangerous and should be treated. It can cause heartbeat to double, signaling trouble for patients with heart ailments.

Aside from the normal physiological mechanisms of fever, there is another important way in which the body heats and cools itself. As a fever sets in and the body begins to generate more heat, muscles contract rapidly to bring on shiver-

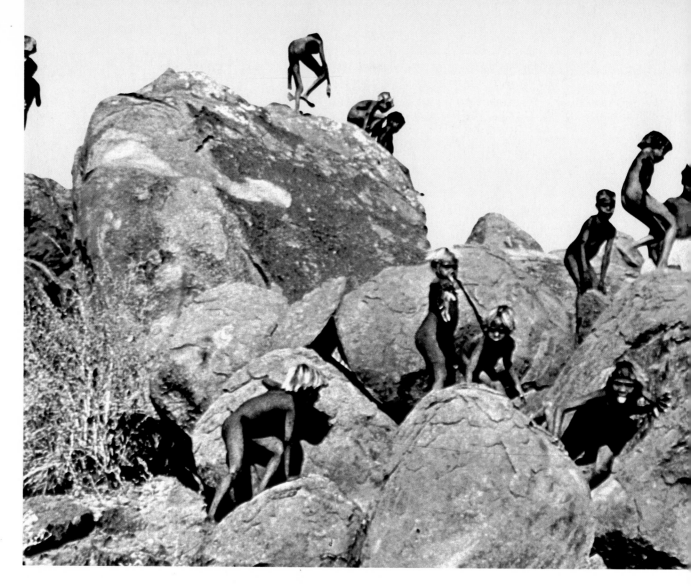

ing and chills. We feel cold and will throw on a sweater or blanket. In this way, our actions aid the body in maintaining temperature. When the body is too cold, we feel uncomfortable. Adding clothing traps additional layers of air next to the skin and decreases loss of heat by convection. A normal layer of clothing can cut heat loss in half. When we feel too warm, we remove clothing, jump in a swimming pool or cool shower or turn on the air conditioning, reinforcing the work of the body's cooling system.

Climate's Effects

Man's relative hairlessness and thin skin indicate that he originated in a warm climate. His ability to protect himself from hostile environments permitted the migration that has populated almost all regions of the earth. Gradually, his body made changes accommodating to new climates. Australian aborigines, who wear little clothing

and tend to sleep in the open, are equipped far better than most humans to withstand cold temperatures. The cause of such a physiological change is difficult to pinpoint, however, because culture is often a greater influence than genetic inheritance. Some Eskimos have a higher than normal metabolism that enables them to heat their bodies in the severe cold of their environment. Their metabolism may be as much as 13 to 33 percent higher than the metabolic rate of people living in a temperate climate. This change is not an inherited physiological adaptation. It is related to the Eskimo's diet, which is high in fish.

Specialized adaptations to heat are more indistinct because all humans, regardless of native climate, are well adapted to surviving in heat, possibly because of man's origins as a tropical animal. People native to hot climates generally have less body fat than those living in cool climates. Body fat insulates and slows heat loss.

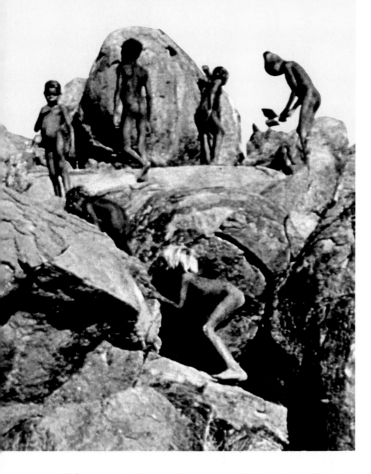

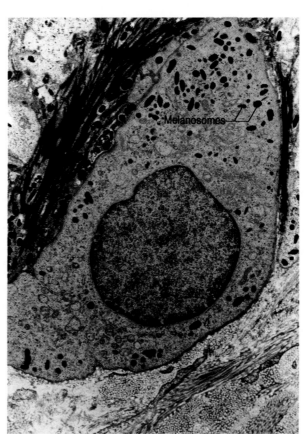

Melanosomes

Tolerance to heat also seems higher in tall, thin people than in short, squat people because the greater body surface enables them to dissipate heat more effectively. Yet there is no strong evidence that natives of desert or tropics inherit a different metabolism. All humans seem equally capable of acclimating to extreme heat.

Man has adapted to changes in climate in another, more pronounced, way. The wide variety of human skin color is a direct measure of the diverse climates man has come to know. All skin color stems from the same substance, melanin. Melanin is the name of a class of pigments widespread throughout nature. The dark blotches that a banana develops in ripening are caused by melanin. The black spots on a leopard's skin also arise from melanin. Two forms of melanin color the skin, hair and eyes of man. The major pigment, eumelanin, produces shades of brown and black. Phaeomelanin is the pigment of red hair.

Skin color, in all its variations, stems from a monochromatic palette, the melanocyte. All human beings have roughly the same number of these cells. The small, dark ovals clustered within the cell are melanosomes, granules of melanin.

71

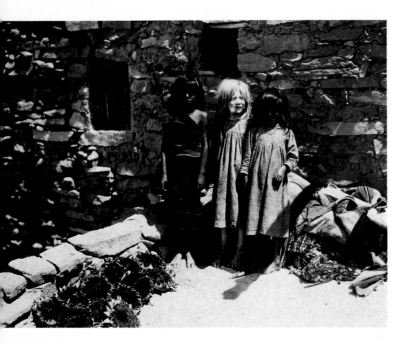

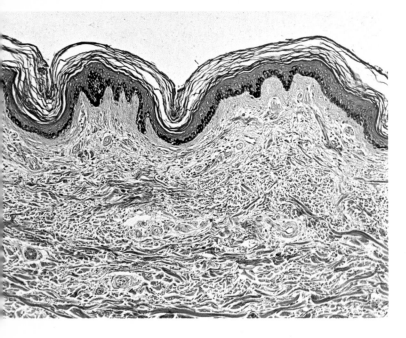

A cross section of skin reveals a thin but rich layer of melanin, stained dark purple, lying between the lighter band of epidermis above, and the mottled dermis below. Dead epidermal cells coat the skin's surface.

Tiny granules of melanin are produced in cells called melanocytes. Melanocytes have the same embryonic origin as nerve cells. They emerge near the tissue that will become the brain, migrate to the skin and come to rest in the deepest layer of the epidermis, usually evenly spaced throughout it.

Pigment production is a continuous process, set into motion by an enzyme called tyrosinase. Melanocytes are spider shaped, with long irregular arms that reach out from the cell body. The arms of each melanocyte link it with about ten surrounding cells. Melanocytes inject pigment granules, melanosomes, into the neighboring cells, thus spreading pigment across the skin. Freckles, a result of the pigment's gathering in clusters, can occur in all skin colors but are most prominent in light skin.

Regardless of skin color, all human beings have the same approximate number of melanocytes in the skin — roughly equivalent to one percent of all skin cells. Differences in skin color are due to the amount of melanin the cells produce. The production of melanin is linked to the pigment's role, which is to protect the body from ultraviolet light, a potentially harmful portion of sunlight.

Light is a form of electromagnetic radiation, a comparatively narrow category in a spectrum that includes radio waves and X-rays. Light falls somewhere between these two, differentiated by the length and frequency of its waves. But visible light, the group of wavelengths we perceive as different colors, is only a portion of the total light spectrum. Visible light is surrounded by invisible light — infrared at one end and ultraviolet at the other.

Skin color represents a compromise between two of the skin's most important functions — provider and protector. Small, steady amounts of ultraviolet radiation are an essential part of the skin's production of vitamin D. In great quantities, however, ultraviolet light turns against the body. Its burning rays can permanently damage body tissues. Ideally, the melanin level maintains a delicate midpoint at which the body receives enough, but not too much, ultraviolet light.

Melanin absorbs ultraviolet rays and converts them into harmless infrared rays. The more melanin in the body the more efficient the absorption and the better the protection. Yet, there is another factor skin must take into account to reach this balance. Ultraviolet light strikes different parts of the Earth in different concentrations. As the sun's radiation passes through the atmosphere, a thin blanket of bluish gas, ozone, filters out many ultraviolet rays. More ultraviolet rays are screened out when light passes through the atmosphere at an angle. Thus, ultraviolet radiation is greatest at the equator, where sunlight is most direct. From the equator toward the poles, ultraviolet radiation diminishes progressively because the sun's rays strike the Earth at greater and greater angles. In order to reach the proper balance between too little and too much ultraviolet light, the amount of melanin in the skin must correspond to the amount of ultraviolet light the skin is regularly exposed to.

No one knows what the skin color of the first humans was. Most scientists believe, however, they were dark-skinned and that light skin emerged later as man migrated to less tropical regions, where colder climates forced him to wear more clothing. The additional layers of clothing, combined with heavily pigmented skin, probably proved too effective a shield against ultraviolet light. Without enough ultraviolet radiation to set vitamin D production in motion, the body would be unable to properly absorb calcium and phosphorus, the minerals that give bone its rigidity. The bones would progressively weaken and buckle under the body's weight, resulting in the characteristic bowlegged look of rickets. The disease also cripples the pelvic bones and can make childbearing difficult or impossible. In this way, natural selection, the gradual process that favors those best suited to their environment, led to the development of light-skinned populations in environments with less ultraviolet radiation.

Had the process been reversed, with light-skinned people moving to a hot, equatorial climate, the amount of melanin in skin would have offered only a limited defense against the burning ultraviolet rays. Gradually, their numbers would have been thinned out, with the greatest survival rate falling to individuals most fit for that environment.

The distribution of light skin in regions that receive little ultraviolet radiation and darker skin in regions that receive more generally holds true around the world. Light-skinned populations inhabit the Northern Hemisphere, with the lightest occurring in northern Europe, where ultraviolet radiation is further restricted by the cloud layers that frequently blanket the area. Light skin is found throughout North America and grows darker in Central and South America. Likewise, it is light in Russia and becomes progressively darker closer to the Mediterranean. Skin color in North Africa is not substantially different from that in southern Europe — a warm, brown color that tans readily. It deepens considerably to the south, particularly along the west coast of Africa and along the valley of the Congo River. These areas are hot but not particularly sunny. The land is heavily forested, and the climate tends to be very humid, with heavy rainfall. Because the people of this region have very dark skin, one would expect that they are exposed to the greatest amount of ultraviolet radiation. That this is not so suggests another factor that may have contributed to the evolution of the variety in skin color. Color may also have served as camouflage for human beings just as it does for many other animals. A sand-colored skin in the desert or dark skin in a dark forest could help make its owner less conspicuous.

There are similar color gradations moving southeast from Europe into the Middle East and India. In Asia, too, northern peoples are lighter skinned, while those in the south, in Vietnam and Indonesia, are darker. Native Australians are also dark-skinned. Like western Africans, their coloring may have developed for the purpose of camouflage as much as for protection from ultraviolet radiation, because ultraviolet radiation is not so great a danger there.

Although skin is said to be red or yellow, there are no such skin colors. North American Indians, Europeans and northern Asians have skin colors that fall in a closely similar range. Indians have skin that tans readily, which may give the impression of a ruddier color. Asians frequently have a yellow cast because the outermost layer of their skin, the stratum corneum, is thicker than

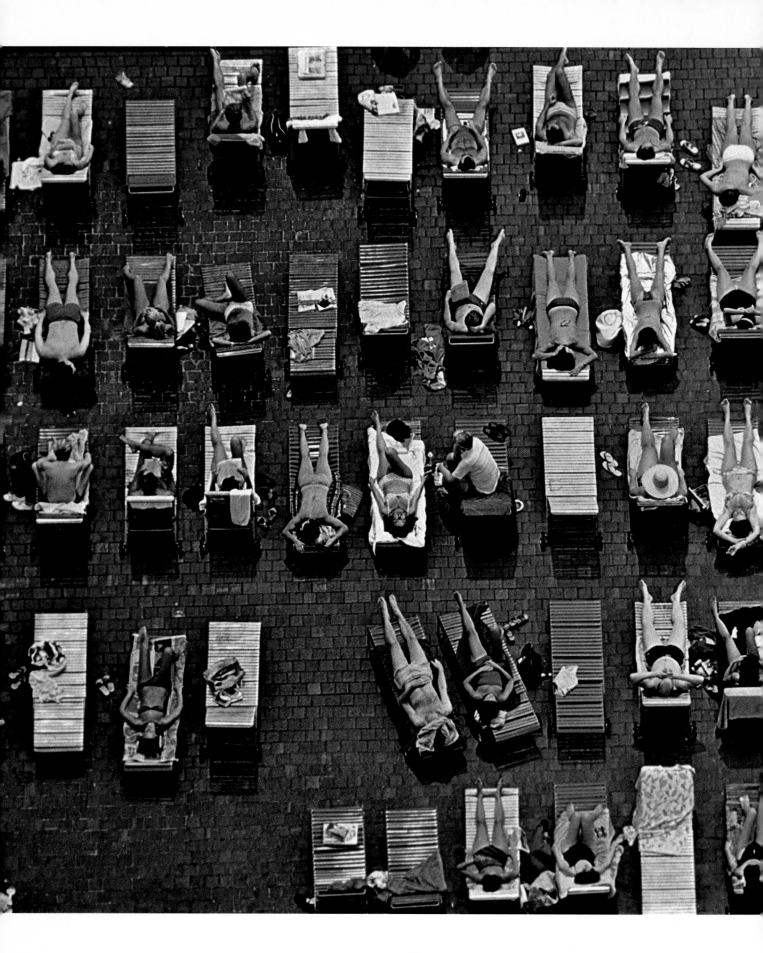

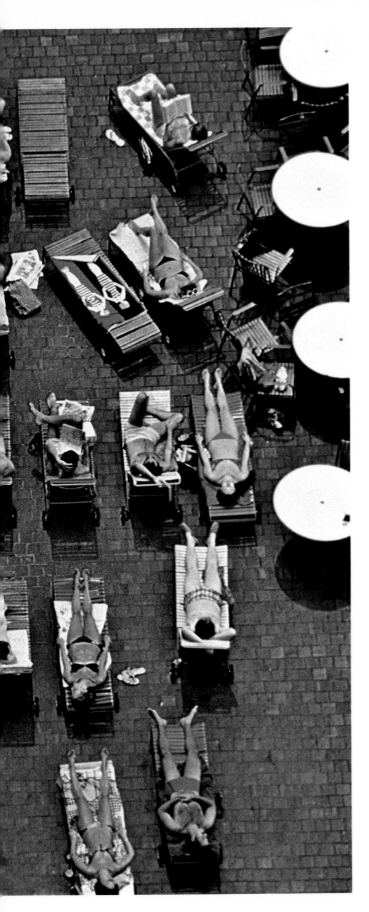

Caucasians'. This layer of cells consists mostly of keratin, which naturally has a yellow or orange tint to it. In each case, the skin probably appears different because of its combination with different racial characteristics such as facial structure.

Today, with world travel a relatively simple and commonplace matter, people with different skin colors live in all parts of the world, apparently wrested from nature's protective boundaries with no ill effects. Yet a number of clues, some subtle, some not, indicate that nature's skin specializations are still very much a working force and that climates to which we are not specially adapted may still be a threat to our health. By the early twentieth century, rickets was still a serious threat to black schoolchildren in parts of the United States. Now that vitamin D is added to milk, the disease has been almost eradicated in both the United States and Europe. But people with light skin still face a grave danger when they live in areas they are not well adapted to, for they run the highest risk of skin cancer.

A Rising Incidence

Skin cancer is the most common form of cancer. Ultraviolet light is its leading cause. People of northern European descent, having the least amounts of melanin, are most prone. Ireland, with a fair-skinned population, has one of the world's highest rates of skin cancer, even though it does not receive especially high amounts of ultraviolet light. Among blacks, the disease is rare.

This form of cancer has been on the rise since the 1940s, when tanned skin came into fashion. For centuries, aristocratic women prided themselves on a lily-white complexion. Tanned skin was the mark of the worker who labored outdoors. Women carefully guarded their faces from the sun with large hats and parasols. But nothing changes if not fashion. With the growing popularity of seaside resorts, sports and other leisure pursuits after World War II, tanned skin became desirable, an enviable vacation souvenir. For those with dark skin, tanning was a relatively harmless pastime. But for light-skinned people, sunbathing became a risk, for they were exposing their skin to amounts of sun nature had not properly equipped them to handle.

75

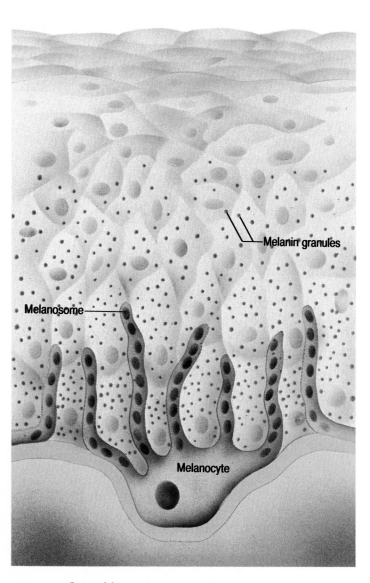

Melanin granules

Melanosome

Melanocyte

Spurred by an increase in ultraviolet radiation, a melanocyte increases its production of melanin. The pigment is injected into neighboring epidermal cells, which begin their steady climb to the surface of the skin. In four to five days, the newly darkened cells reach the surface. The result of all this activity — what we call a sun tan — protects the skin from additional sun damage.

The first result of overexposure to the sun is sunburn, that painful red glow that persists for a few hours to a few days after sunning. The redness comes from an increased blood flow to the area, the skin's way of speeding healing, and from toxic substances released from damaged cells. In response to increased ultraviolet radiation, the skin begins to develop a tan. Tanning is a defense against additional damage. Stimulated by the ultraviolet radiation, melanocytes begin to produce more melanin. Around the melanocytes, cell division increases as the body attempts to repair its tissues. These new cells begin their trip to the surface of the skin, normally a three-to-four-week journey. But the rapid production of new cells speeds up the process, so that the cells reach the surface in only four to five days. Older cells, meanwhile, are shed more quickly than usual, which is why the skin peels after it is sunburned.

It is ironic that tanned skin is associated with a youthful, healthy look. Sun damage is cumulative and irreversible. Steady tanning can lead to premature wrinkles, sags and discoloration. Once the skin is so affected, no amount of facials or moisturizers can reverse the damage, which usually does not show up until later in life.

More serious, skin cancer, like all cancers, produces abnormal cells that grow quickly and unceasingly. If not controlled, they eventually invade other sites. Although the sun is a factor in the development of skin cancer, scientists are not sure how it begins. They suspect the ultraviolet rays cause cell mutations by interfering with a cell's genetic material. Usually, sun-injured cells can repair themselves but those that cannot make repairs may survive with genetic mutations that lead to skin cancer.

There are three main types of skin cancer. The two most common are named for the skin cells in which they occur. Basal cell cancer occurs in the deepest layer of the epidermis. It usually appears as pale, waxy gray nodules or distinct red, scaly patches, but it may take other forms, as well. Squamous cell cancer occurs in the upper layers of the epidermis. It is generally characterized by rough, scaly patches but, like basal cell cancer, can differ greatly in appearance. Basal cell cancer is more frequent but it is less likely to spread and

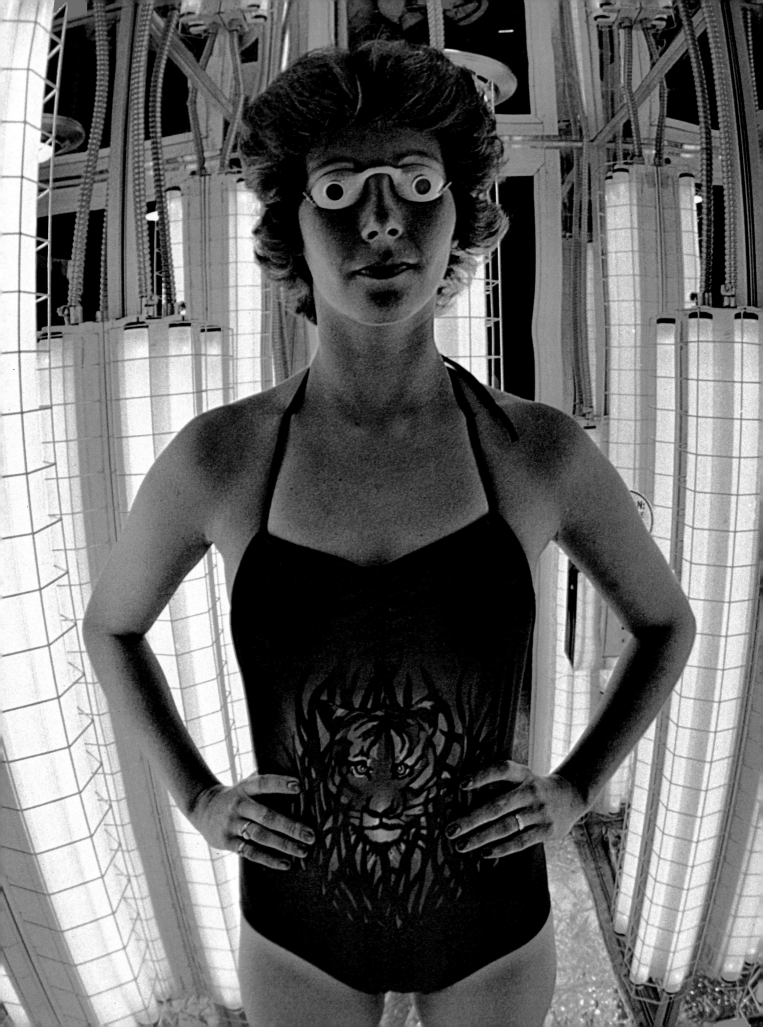

Percivall Pott

Surgeon to the Sweeps

In protecting its owner from vagaries of the environment, skin opens itself up to a multitude of dangers. But skin's superficiality also makes it a measure of health. A disease afflicting it can be seen. It is not surprising that skin was the focus of one of the earliest studies of cancer. The investigator was Percivall Pott, an eighteenth-century surgeon.

In 1729, fifteen-year-old Pott became an apprentice to a surgeon. For seven years, Pott prepared dissection specimens for his master, who lectured on anatomy as well as surgery. By the age of thirty-five, the apprentice succeeded his teacher as full surgeon at London's St. Bartholomew's Hospital. But he did not begin writing the treatises that made him famous until the age of forty-three, when an accident left him with time on his hands.

While riding to work one winter morning, Pott fell from his horse and suffered a compound fracture of the leg. Realizing the seriousness of his condition, he sent two men to find a pair of poles. In the meantime, he arranged to purchase a door. When the men returned, they nailed the poles to the door and carried Pott on the makeshift stretcher to his home. A colleague who examined the leg said it should be

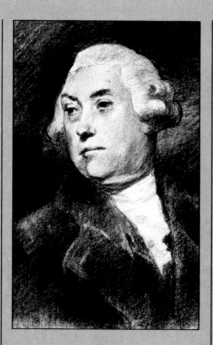

amputated. Pott consented. Just as the instruments were being prepared, however, Pott's old teacher arrived. He looked at the leg and declared that it could be saved. Pott's long confinement was fruitful. While the leg mended, he wrote a treatise on fractures. One type of fracture of the lower leg still bears his name.

Pott practiced medicine when surgery was still in the hands of the knife-wielding barber and quack apothecary who, a contemporary wrote, filled "a physician's prescription though he had not in his shop one medicine mentioned in it." Pott, incensed by such

practices, had no patience with those "who lie in wait to avail themselves of the weaknesses of the infirm and fearful."

Pott felt compassion for his patients. The lives of young chimney sweeps moved him to write in 1775, "The fate of these people seems singularly hard . . . they are thrust up narrow, and sometimes hot chimnies, where they are bruised, burned, and almost suffocated; and when they get to puberty, become peculiarly liable to a most noisome, painful, and fatal disease."

Because the malady often appeared at puberty, doctors treated it as a venereal disease. Chimney sweeps, however, had a rough notion of its true origin, for they called it a "soot wart." It was cancer, Pott concluded, caused by an accumulation of soot in the skin of the scrotum. Having seen the fast and deadly spread of the disease, he recommended quick removal of the diseased tissue.

Pott's finding may well mark the beginning of modern cancer research, for he had identified the first known carcinogen. His modest, 800-word paper carried no sense of its own importance. Of his life's work, he reflected, "My light is almost extinguished. . . . I hope it has burned for the benefit of others."

*Melanocytes, plump ovals when
normal, take on sinister shapes
when stricken with cancer. These,
from a malignant melanoma, the
most threatening of the skin cancers,
are magnified 160 times.*

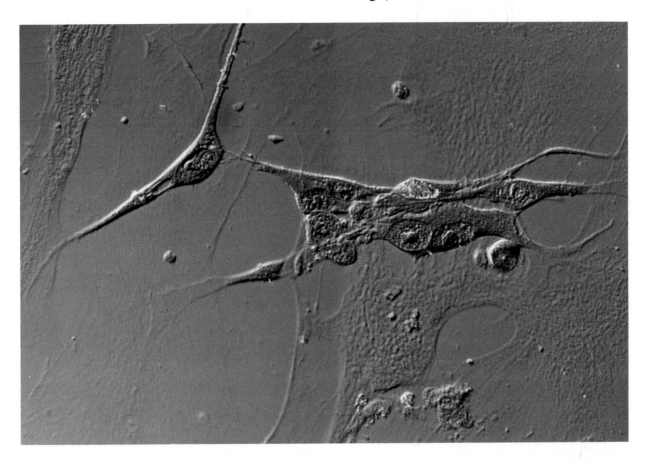

grows more slowly. The third type of skin cancer is more rare but much more virulent. Malignant melanomas usually appear as dark brown or black patches much like moles. They may also develop from moles. Although most skin cancers are not serious or life threatening and can be quickly and easily treated, it is still preferable to prevent them entirely. The best way to do this is to safeguard the body from ultraviolet radiation. The best protection, aside from avoiding the sun altogether, is to avoid it when it is most intense, from about 10:00 A.M. to 3:00 P.M. Sun screens are available in a variety of strengths. The most effective sun screens contain the chemical agent para-aminobenzoic acid, PABA, which duplicates the action of melanin by absorbing ultraviolet rays. Products such as baby oil and coconut butter do not protect the skin from burning at all. And no tanning product, despite commercial claims, hastens the tanning process.

Any new or unusual skin growth should be inspected by a doctor to determine whether or not it is cancerous. If there is any doubt, he will take a sample for microscopic testing. Generally, removal of the growth is all the treatment necessary. Electrosurgery is a technique using an electric current to destroy cancer cells. Cryosurgery destroys the cells by freezing them. The basal and squamous varieties have the highest rate of recovery. Malignant melanomas are more of a threat, for they can quickly spread elsewhere.

Ninety-five percent of skin cancer patients are completely free of cancer following treatment. The success rate is attributable to the ease with which skin cancer can be detected. The skin usually heals quickly after treatment and, in doing so, demonstrates its remarkable regenerative power. A small scar may remain but this, too, is another aspect of our versatile body covering. The skin is a living record of experience.

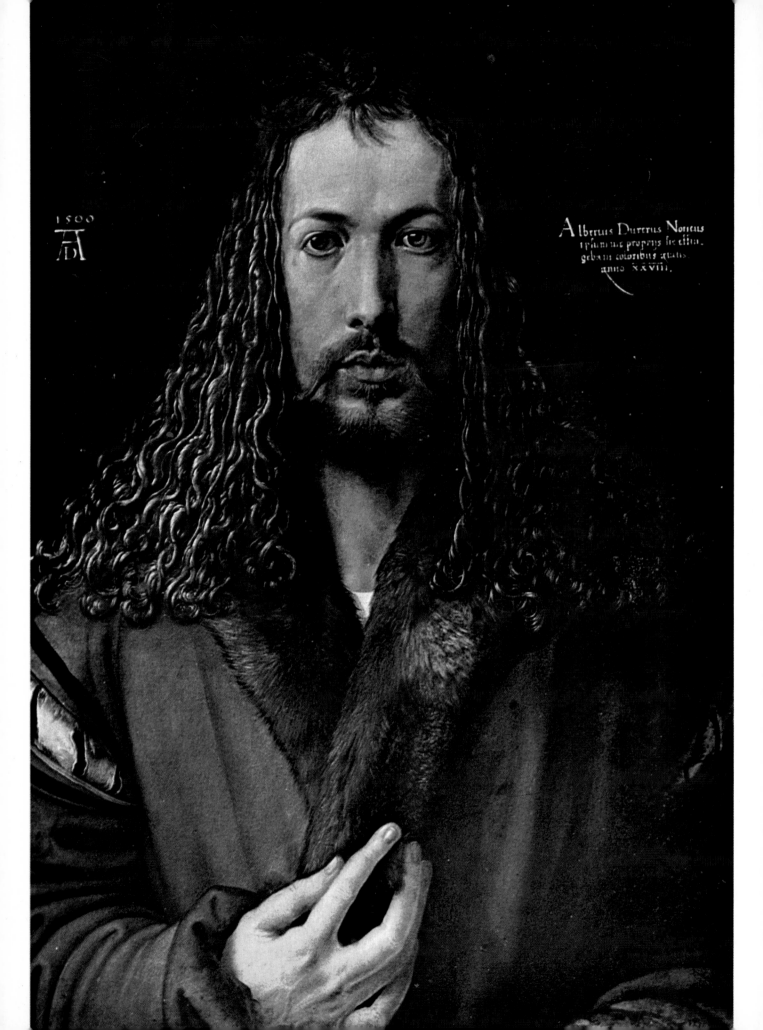

1500

AD

Albertus Durerus Noricus
ipſum me propriis ſic effin-
gebam coloribus ætatis
anno XXVIII.

Chapter 4

Finery on the Fabric

Sometimes called the naked ape, man is, strictly speaking, neither naked nor an ape. Human beings have roughly as many hairs per square inch of skin as monkeys, chimps and gorillas. Except on the scalp, under the arms and in the genital region, however, most body hair is fine, all but invisible to the naked eye and not nearly thick enough to hide the skin. As man became differentiated from the apes through the slow stages of evolution, he gradually lost the hair that once covered his body. Why our species, *Homo sapiens,* abandoned its thick pelt is a question that still puzzles anthropologists.

Hair is actually a specialized form of skin, as are hooves, scales, claws, horns and feathers. In one guise or another, skin forms the exterior of virtually every animal. Feathers bring warmth, waterproofing and flight to birds. Scales are the armor of reptiles and fish. From the aardvark to the zebra, hooves and claws aid both fight and flight. Hair, unique to mammals, makes up the tiger's stripes, and in a modified form, the porcupine's quills and the horn of the rhinoceros. A species of algae lives in the hair of the three-toed sloth, turning the animal's coat a light shade of green that helps camouflage it in the tree tops. Man's paltry coat, however, provides no camouflage, defense or weaponry and little warmth.

Man's hairlessness is a mystery because it does not appear to confer an obvious evolutionary advantage. Anthropologists and other scientists have proposed many explanations for the gradual molt of *Homo sapiens*. As man's ancestors began to capitalize on their evolving intelligence, the discoveries of clothing and fire may have made hair expendable. Hair may have hindered facial expressions of anger, fear and affection. Exposing the skin for the sake of communication might have proved more valuable than covering it for protection. One imaginative theory suggests that man underwent an aquatic phase at some point

Over the centuries, in many cultures, hair has symbolized strength, beauty, inspiration and divinity. German painter and engraver Albrecht Dürer painted his Self-Portrait *of 1500 in reverent imitation of Christ, says art historian Erwin Panofsky. Dürer's profusion of carefully arranged curls frames an almost otherworldly expression. His self-portrait embodies both a man of the Renaissance and the mystery of the Christian savior.*

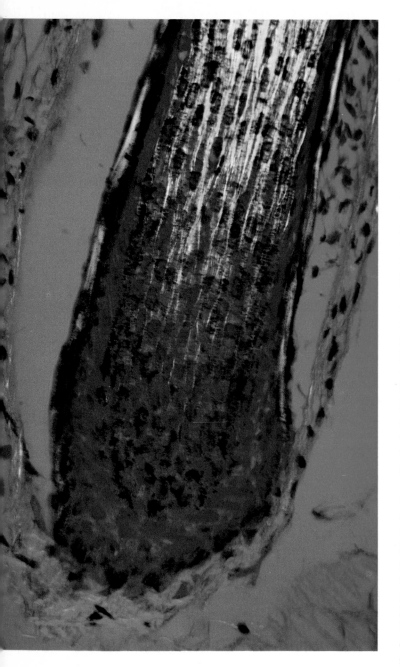

A hair follicle sliced thin shows cells at the base of a hair packed tightly together and speckled with cell nuclei and deposits of melanin. Melanin colors the hair; the nuclei gradually harden and disappear.

in his evolutionary history. Like dolphins and whales, which are also mammals, man might have lost his pelt to glide more easily through the water. Among the primates, only man possesses a layer of fat beneath the skin to insulate him from the cold, just as a whale's blubber keeps out the ocean's chill. This theory also suggests that chimpanzees dread being in the water but man does not because it was man's natural habitat in millennia gone by.

A Hunter Without Hair

Most scientists, however, believe that hirsute man was at a disadvantage as a hunter in the tropical sun. As a result, he lost his hair over many generations. The diet of early man — nuts, roots, birds, lizards and small mammals — probably required nearly continual motion. Because food was scattered, our ancestors may have maintained a steady trot for many hours in search of prey. They probably foraged during the heat of the day to avoid competition with nocturnal predators such as the lion and leopard. To keep cool during the chase, two changes would have served man well — the loss of hair and the development of numerous sweat glands. Man's cooling system has become, over time, the most efficient of any mammal's, in part because his skin is not covered by thick, matted hair.

The hair that remains on man serves a few useful purposes. Eyebrows keep sweat out of the eyes, and eyelashes warn the eyelids to close if dust or insects get dangerously near. Tiny hairs in the ears and nostrils filter out airborne particles. Hair of the armpits helps reduce friction during walking and running; pubic hair may serve the same purpose during sexual intercourse. Hair also contributes to the sense of touch. Beneath the skin, each hair is encircled by the endings of a nerve. Any movement of the hair sends an impulse to the brain. Extraordinarily sensitive hairs called vibrissae help dogs, cats and many other mammals feel their way through the world. The whiskers that surround a dog's mouth are vibrissae. Squirrels have these sensory hairs on their abdomens, lemurs on their wrists.

Because man has lost so much hair, many people have wondered why he has any left at all.

Some scientists suspect that man is evolving toward complete hairlessness — the intelligent ape, bald and bare. Since the hair on the human head offers scant protection and little warmth, they reason that a layer of fat beneath the skin might do just as well. After all, millions of men around the world have lost almost all the hair on their heads without any ill effects. Although they serve no obvious purpose, pubic hair and axillary hair, the hair of the armpits, have subtle uses. Appearing at puberty, they are visible signs of sexual maturity.

The pubic and axillary regions also contain apocrine glands, modified sweat glands. These glands secrete a fluid that exudes a noticeable odor when it encounters air and some common bacteria on the skin. Scientists know that the distinctive odors of many animals play an important role in sexual attraction. Human scent, too, has a role in romance. Pubic and axillary hair trap these apocrine secretions and foster their fragrance. The secretions are, in part, what makes human beings smell human. Beards, mustaches and body hair in men are probably epigamic, or related to sexual dominance. Many species of monkeys have beards, mustaches and shaggy manes that serve to intimidate their rivals. Facial and body hair may persist in human males for the same reason.

All of this hair, whatever its purpose, sprouts from tiny tunnels called follicles. Follicles are narrow indentations of the outer layer of skin, the epidermis. They begin to appear in the skin of the fetus about three months after conception, in a pattern that suggests reptilian scales. By three months before birth, we have all the follicles we are ever going to have. The follicles produce a soft, downy fuzz called lanugo that covers the fetus evenly from head to toe. Before birth, vellus hair, a lightly pigmented down, replaces lanugo. On the scalp, vellus hair later gives way to terminal, or mature, hair. Vellus hair and terminal hair can sprout alternately from the same follicle. Before puberty, boys have vellus hair on their faces. The influence of hormones at puberty signals the follicles to start producing the terminal hair of beards. On careful scrutiny, a man's bald head proves not to be bald at all. Terminal

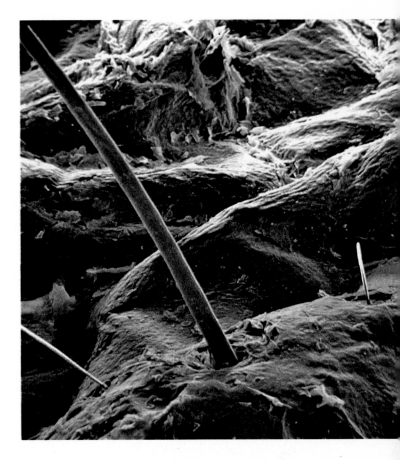

Like the trunk of a lone palm on a parched landscape, a mature hair arches upward from the skin of a woman's calf. Small, lightly pigmented vellus hairs sprout from the skin on either side of the hair. Vellus hair is almost invisible to the naked eye.

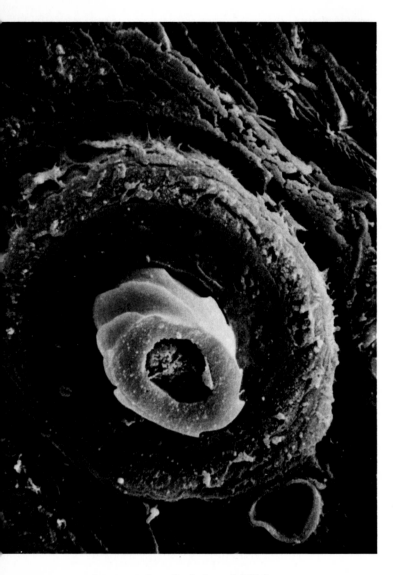

A cross section of a hair and follicle shows the dark central medulla of the hair, the whiter ring of the cortex and the scales of the cuticle emerging from the hair like spiral blades. The two rings of tissue surrounding the hair form the root sheath. Strands of connective tissue cling like cobwebs to the outside of the sheath.

hairs have dropped out and left the vellus variety in their place.

To create a follicle, a small pocket of the epidermis burrows into the underlying layer of skin, the dermis. Within this protected pouch, the follicle builds a hair. The hair itself consists of the root, the portion inside the follicle, and the shaft, which protrudes above the skin. The outermost layer of the follicle is part of the dermis and made of connective tissue. Inside are several layers of epidermal cells that make up the root sheath. A collar of nerve endings from a single nerve encircles the follicle about halfway between its base and the surface of the skin. The nerve endings signal the brain if the hair is touched. A small cluster of sebaceous glands drains into every hair follicle, coating the hair with sebum, a mixture of fats, oils, soaps, cell fragments and a few other ingredients. Sebum lubricates and protects the hair.

Small strands of smooth muscle, the arrector pili, also attach to the follicle. Cold or fright makes this muscle contract, and its contraction pulls the follicle bolt upright, creating a small bump on the surface of the skin. Commonly known as goose bumps or goose flesh, the condition is usually temporary, but not always. When British troops were driven off the European mainland at Dunkirk in the early months of World War II, some soldiers were so haunted that their hair stood on end for months. British army doctor Sir Arthur Hurst reported that the horror of trench warfare in World War I left some soldiers in a permanent state of terror. The hair of their heads and bodies, wrote Hurst, remained persistently on end.

Hair itself is nothing more than dead skin packed in a column. It grows from the bottom of the root upward. The papilla, a small cone of dermal tissue rich in blood vessels, protrudes into the base of the follicle to nourish a layer of epidermal cells known as the hair matrix. The cells of the matrix rapidly reproduce and die. As the pressure of new cells appearing behind them drives them up the follicle, they flatten, elongate and bind together to form the hair. A mature hair looks something like a scallion, with a long, thin shaft sprouting from a small bulb. Dying cells

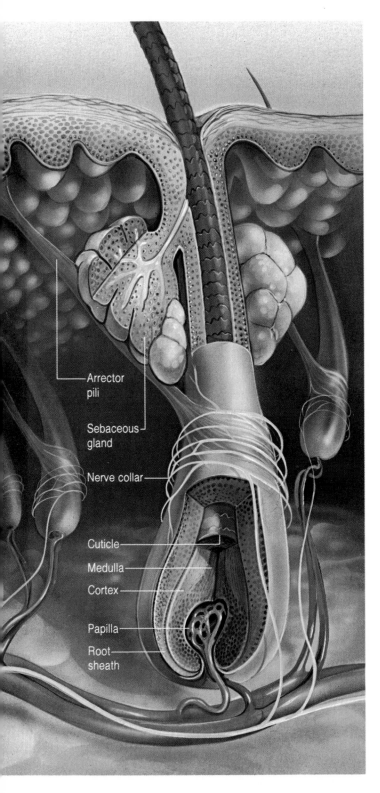

A hair follicle is a cylinder of epidermal cells that have tunneled into the underlying dermis. Blood vessels bring nourishment at the papilla. Muscle, nerve and sebaceous glands adjoin every follicle.

Arrector pili

Sebaceous gland

Nerve collar

Cuticle

Medulla

Cortex

Papilla

Root sheath

from the matrix produce keratin, a tough, insoluble protein that is the major constituent of hair, nails and the outermost layer of skin. Three layers of keratinized cells form every hair. The outer sheath, or cuticle, of hair is made of cells arranged in overlapping scales. The cuticle encircles the narrow, elongated cells of the cortex, the middle layer. The core of the hair is the medulla, a column of cells shaped like cubes and interspersed with small air pockets.

The development of fingernails and toenails proceeds in much the same way. Nails consist of a root and a body. The root, about one-third of the nail, is hidden beneath the skin. Beneath the root lies a layer of cells called the nail matrix. As in hair, cells of the matrix rapidly reproduce, die and become tough scales of keratin that cement together to form the nail. The rich blood supply of the nail bed produces a pink color. Air pockets at the base of the thumbnail and some of the fingernails leave a pale crescent lunula, or "little moon." In the fetus, nails begin to form in the fifth month after conception.

Genes That Color Hair

The color of hair, like that of skin, depends on melanin, dark pigment manufactured by melanocytes and deposited in growing hairs. Most of the pigment in a hair resides in the cortex. The subtleties of hair color come from light reflecting off oils on the surface of the hair, pigment in the cortex, unpigmented bits of the medulla and tiny pockets of air within the shaft. If the pigment has disappeared, hair looks gray or white.

The amount of melanin in a hair — and the resulting color — is genetically determined. Genes that govern hair color sometimes take a few years to make their true nature known. Towheaded children often become brunet adults. A rich deposit of melanin makes hair dark brown or black. Smaller endowments yield brown, sandy-colored and blond hair. Red hair seems to be the product of a separate gene. This gene produces an independent red pigment that simply adds to other colors in a person's hair. Dark hair obscures the red pigment. When the pigment is mixed with light hair, the result is strawberry blond. True redheads possess only the special red pigment.

Pockets of pigment in the core, or medulla, of a hair and more uniform deposits of pigment in the surrounding cortex give hair its color. In a gray hair, below, air replaces pigment.

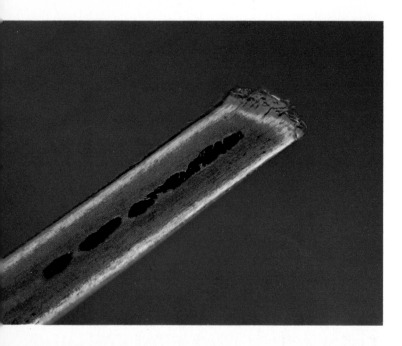

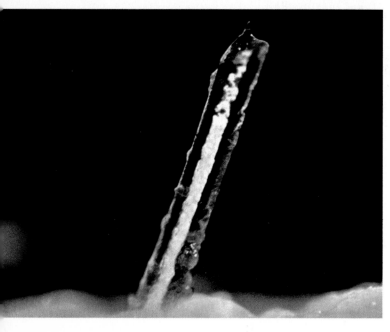

Anthropologist Ashley Montagu notes that the absence of the darker melanin pigment in redheads seems to have consequences besides red hair. Redheads are even more prone to sunburn than blonds. When some redheads suffer severe burns from extreme heat or fires, they take an unusually long time to heal, and their wounds often form thick, raised scars called keloids. The blood of some redheads, Montagu says, is comparatively slow to clot and some seem to require greater amounts of anesthetics and lower doses of radiation than other patients.

The shape and size of hair follicles determine the shape and texture of hair. Straight hair follicles grow straight hairs, but bowed follicles yield curly hair. In cross section, straight hair tends to be round, curly hair flat or oval. The number of active follicles per square inch determines whether hair is thick or thin. Coarseness and fineness describe the diameter of the hair itself.

To the delight of hairdressers, the shape of an individual hair can be changed. Permanents temporarily break some of the chemical bonds that determine a hair's shape. Altered in this way, a hair can be wrapped around a roller or wound in a tight spiral and allowed to rebuild its chemical scaffolding. Until it is replaced by new growth, the hair will hold its new shape. Intense heat can also dissolve chemical bonds, enabling those who so desire to iron their curly hair straight. To a limited degree, water works the same way. Wet curls relax slightly, and rewind as they dry.

The arrival of uninvited gray hairs persuades many people to try hair coloring. No one knows why the cells that manufacture pigment for hair wind down over the years. Melanocytes in the skin last a lifetime and sometimes even step up the production of pigment with age. Hair cannot turn white overnight, although for hundreds of years people have chosen to believe it could. The grief of Shah Jahan of India at the death of his wife, Mumtaz Mahal, supposedly bleached his hair pure white. In her memory, he built a tomb, the magnificent Taj Mahal. It is said that the beard and hair of Sir Thomas More, chancellor under Henry VIII, turned white on the eve of his execution. Whether it was white or not, More's beard was in his thoughts at the end. He lifted it from under his chin as he placed his head on the block, saying "This hath not offended the king." Although they lived two centuries apart and on different sides of the English Channel, both Mary, Queen of Scots, and Marie Antoinette, Queen of France, allegedly developed white hair on the eve of their executions. The Scottish Mary often wore wigs, however, so her sudden loss of hair color might have been more of a revelation than a transformation. Contemporary accounts reveal that Marie Antoinette's hair had turned white long before her death. The absence of hair dyes and a hairdresser in prison is a more likely explanation of the whiteness of her hair than the fear she may have felt on the day she was to face the guillotine.

Because the loss of pigmented hair leaves only gray behind, hair can indeed present the appearance of quickly turning white. One variety of baldness, alopecia areata, attacks pigmented hair almost exclusively. This disease may be responsible for many tales of overnight blanching, but it usually takes weeks or months for the hair to change colors. Often, the hair that fills in after attacks of alopecia areata is a shining white.

Graying is part of hair's normal pattern of growth. Between 100,000 and 150,000 hairs blanket the head. At any moment, about 90 percent of them are growing and the other 10 percent resting. Individual hairs grow for two to six years and then rest for about three months. At the end of the cycle, often to the dismay of their owners, they drop out. Everyone loses between 30 and 100 hairs every day, but they are continually replaced by an equal number. As people age, more of the replacement hairs are gray.

Cells of the scalp replenish themselves in a pattern similar to that of hair, but they supplant one another more rapidly. The skin of the head renews itself about once a month. When the rate of this regeneration becomes unusually rapid, the dead skin cells begin to flake and dandruff results. The cause of dandruff still eludes dermatologists, but medicated shampoos can usually keep it under control.

Hair grows at different rates on different parts of the body and at different ages. Women between the ages of sixteen and twenty-four have

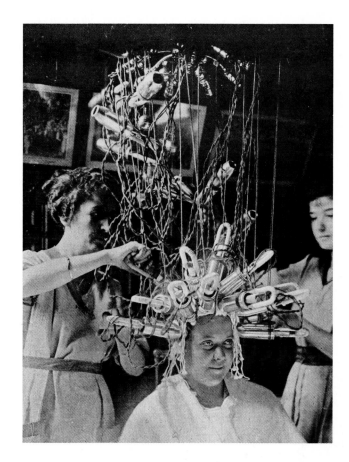

Hair can be colored, frizzed, straightened, curled and treated in many other ungentle ways. Early in the twentieth century, Karl Nessler invented this machine to give hair permanent waves.

The microscopist's stain makes a cluster of hair follicles look like pools of color in an abstract painting. A head of hair on a human being consists of roughly 150,000 hairs, although the number varies with age and from person to person. Hair grows about one-half inch per month. Follicles work independently of each other, each growing a hair on its own schedule. A follicle of the scalp labors for two to six years on a hair, rests for a few months, sheds the hair and begins again. Uncut, the average human hair would not grow beyond about three feet in length.

the fastest-growing hair. On the average, hair grows about thirteen one-thousandths of an inch a day or almost a half-inch per month, diminishing slightly with age. At this rate, hair six years old would be about three feet long if left uncut. Twenty-five feet of hair represents a lifetime of labor for the scalp. People with exceptionally long hair have been featured in circuses for years. The seven Sutherland sisters, one of the attractions of the Barnum and Bailey circus in the 1880s, had, among them, hair that was thirty-six feet, ten inches long, or about five feet apiece. India's Swami Pandarasannadhi, the head of a monastery, was reported to possess twenty-six feet of hair in 1949, the most luxuriant growth of hair ever recorded.

Fingernails grow more slowly than hair, about one-tenth of an inch a month, but they grow continuously throughout life. For reasons unknown, nails grow more slowly in infancy, old age and winter. Unclipped, they loop into spirals like the horns of a ram. According to the *Guinness Book of World Records*, Shridhar Chillal of India has the world's longest nails. One hundred eight and one-half inches of keratin spiral out from the fingers of his left hand. His left thumbnail alone is twenty-seven and one-half inches long.

Contrary to many a yarn, fingernails and hair cannot grow after death. The skin of the scalp, face and fingers sometimes contracts slightly in death, so a corpse neatly trimmed and clean-shaven at a funeral may look a bit bristly later on. Macabre tales of exhumed coffins filled with flowing hair or foot-long beards on men who were beardless in life are shaggy horror stories and nothing more.

A lack of hair in this life, rather than its abundance after death, is a common fear of mortal man. Baldness afflicts more than twenty million Americans. Two-thirds of American men aged sixty-five and over show signs of baldness. Through history, countless lotions, potions and incantations have been used to combat it. Six thousand years ago, one queen mother of Egypt recommended rubbing the scalp with an ointment sure to shock new spirit into malingering follicles. The ingredients included toes of a dog, refuse of dates and the hoof of an ass. Egyptians

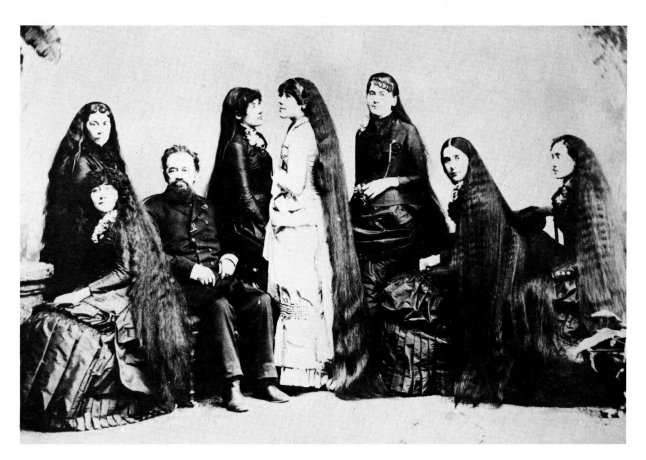

also rubbed fat over the scalp to restore hair. A recipe for a salve called for fat from a lion, hippopotamus, crocodile, cat, serpent and Egyptian goat. Romans sought such restorative powers from bear's fat. Dioscorides, a first-century Greek physician, advised that baldness could be prevented by twice-weekly treatments of the broth of vipers boiled alive. Scalp rubs have shown little promise, but the search continues. Minoxidil, a drug first prescribed for high blood pressure, has caused hair to grow from balding scalps as an unexpected side effect. Tests on the drug's effectiveness as a scalp rub are under way.

X-rays, burns, chemotherapy, diseases, high fever, emotional trauma, pregnancy and oral contraceptives can all be hard on hair. Alopecia areata and other diseases of the scalp can cause diffuse, or patchy, hair loss. In severe cases, these diseases can lead to complete loss of hair over the body. But the most common cause of baldness is what dermatologists call androgenetic alopecia, or male-pattern baldness. No medicine known to science can stop or even slow the process. It usually begins with a receding hairline and a small thin spot on the crown. Gradually, they grow toward each other and merge. A horseshoe of healthy hair stretching from temple to temple

above the ears remains. In women, androgenetic alopecia most often takes the form of a mild thinning at the crown. Common baldness is simply a part of human growth. The same hormones that trigger the growth of terminal hairs beneath the arms and in the pubic area prompt the loss of some terminal hairs in the scalp. Eunuchs of the royal oriental courts lacked these hormones and never went bald.

Hair Repair

Wigs and toupees have hidden the bald truth for thousands of years, but hairpieces have always had drawbacks. Cheap wigs do not look like real hair. All hairpieces must be firmly secured to the head with hairpins, glue, tape or some other adhesive. Many are hot and require at least as much care as normal hair. They can sometimes wiggle off. In recent decades, hair weaving and hair implants have offered a partial solution to baldness and wigs, but they are not completely satisfactory. Hair weaving entails tying a hairpiece to remaining strands of hair on a balding head. Properly woven, the hairpiece stays attached during the most strenuous work or play. But the living cords that anchor the hairpiece grow at their usual pace. In a few weeks or

89

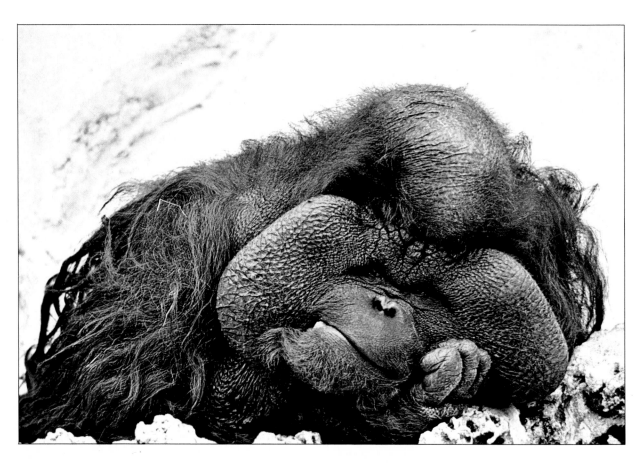

Man is not alone in his baldness. Other primates, like this melancholy orangutan, the ouakari and the stump-tailed macaque, also succumb to the effects of aging as the years rob them of hair.

months, the hairpiece is loose and the weaver must tend to the fabric again. To solve this problem, some hair clinics have resorted to hair implants. In this procedure, a physician carves small tunnels under the scalp and loops a piece of flexible teflon or surgical thread through the tunnel. By law, only a physician can perform this procedure. After the loops are in place, hairdressers or other hair specialists tie the hairpiece to the loops. Because the loops do not grow, the hairpiece remains tight, but some customers develop pain and infections.

A third alternative to wigs and toupees is the hair transplant. With a circular surgical tool called a trephine, a physician cuts small plugs of bald scalp from the top of the head and replaces them with hairy plugs from the back or sides of the head. Each plug is about three-eighths of an inch in diameter, although the size can vary. Small scabs quickly form over the plugs and drop off after a week or two, often taking transplanted hairs with them. These hairs, however, are not the object of the operation. Hair transplants might more accurately be called scalp transplants, since healthy follicles from the back of the head are moved forward. For about three months, the follicles remain dormant in a kind of transplant shock, but after adapting to their new homes, they begin to produce new hair. In nine months, a crown once bald can show a respectable thatch of hair. But the procedure is costly and not every patient is happy with his new growth.

Most men simply choose to live with their baldness. In spite of jokes about frostbitten or sunburned scalps, bald men gain a certain respect accorded to age. As a thick shock of black hair and a hairy chest are signs of vigor and virility, a smooth pate symbolizes maturity, intelligence and wisdom. Man is not alone in having a hairless dome. Orangutans, stump-tailed macaques and the ouakari, a species of monkey, all grow bald as they grow old. In the human imagination, baldness is often seen as a step of evolutionary advancement. In films and literature, visitors from other planets or even from mankind's own future all have shining heads.

Perhaps one reason why so many people fear baldness is that abundant hair has long symbolized power, strength, virility and beauty. Greek, Roman, Assyrian, Hindu and Egyptian cultures have all worshiped sun gods blessed with golden, flowing hair. The Toltecs of Mexico, who flourished in about 1000 A.D., called their sun god Quetzalcoatl, or "bushy-haired." The Assyrian god-hero Gilgamesh, the model for Hercules, Samson and other mythical heroes, was a long-hair. The waning of the sun's powers, in fall and winter, was seen as a kind of celestial haircut in some cultures. Even today, on the Isle of Skye off the coast of Scotland, one name for the sun is "grugach," which means hairy.

The biblical muscle man Samson confided to his faithless lover Delilah that "there hath not been a razor upon mine head . . . from my mother's womb: if I am shaven, then my strength will go from me, and I shall become weak, and be like any other man." After he fell asleep in Delilah's lap, she called in a servant to shave his seven

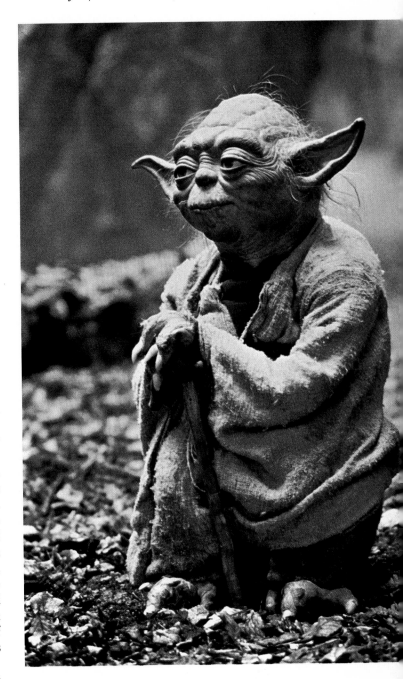

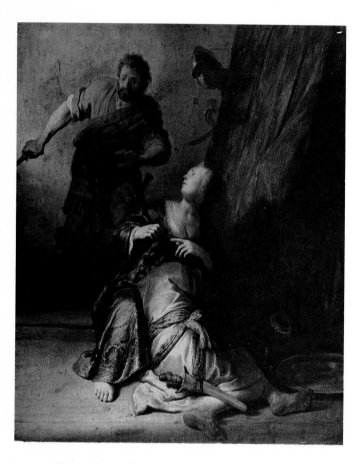

Having learned the secret of his strength and lulled him to sleep in her lap, Samson's lover Delilah calls for a servant to cut off his hair. The painting is Rembrandt's Samson Betrayed by Delilah.

locks and then delivered him to his enemies, the Philistines. Just as Samson's betrayal illustrates hair's symbolic importance, his ultimate revenge demonstrates its resilience. Samson's hair grew back, and the strength it returned to him enabled him to destroy his enemies. Similarly, some folk tales hold that, as the sun's hair is shorn in winter, it grows again in spring.

Women's hair, in a different way, has always held as much power as men's. In his first letter to the Corinthians, the apostle Paul wrote, "If a woman have long hair, it is a glory unto her." In this glory lie great power and danger. The beautiful hair of Medusa, a Greek maiden, became the source of her persecution. She committed a terrible sacrilege by yielding to the advances of the god Poseidon in the temple of Athena, the virgin goddess of wisdom and art. To punish the vain Medusa and prevent her from attracting another suitor, Athena transformed her hair into a nest of writhing snakes. One look at Medusa turned a man to stone. In German legend, a beautiful maiden called the Lorelei sings on the banks of the Rhine while combing her long tresses. If a passing boatman lets his attention drift from the water before him, he is lost. Mermaids possess the same fatal allure.

Hair's erotic appeal spans the centuries. Australian aborigines prized the clippings of their wives' hair as perhaps their most valuable possession. English engraver William Hogarth wrote in 1753, "One lock of hair falling across the temples has an effect too alluring to be strictly decent." To this day, some orthodox Jewish women show their hair only to their husbands.

Saving the Shavings

The power of witches and wizards was long thought to reside in their hair. Witches on trial in the Middle Ages often had their heads shaved. The shearing sometimes brought forth a confession when the most horrible tortures would not. The notorious inquisitor of fifteenth-century Germany, Jacob Sprenger, sometimes freed witches after shaving them, believing them stripped of their powers. In many cultures of both the East and West, shorn locks and clipped nails were saved, buried or burned to keep them from falling into the hands of witches and sorcerers, who might use them to work black magic against their previous owners. Some people still keep a lock of hair from each of their children as a family heirloom. The superstition began in the ancient belief that preserving a lock of hair from a baby's head would protect the child it came from and ensure a long life.

Hair figures in countless legends. In Europe, red hair was once considered a sign of deceitfulness and treachery. Christianity's greatest betrayer, Judas Iscariot, supposedly had red hair. Europeans believed that if birds built nests out of someone's hair, that person would suffer from headaches and possibly go mad. The phrase "the hair of the dog that bit you" recommends taking a drink to cure a hangover. Its origins lie in the superstition that a dog bite could be healed by rubbing the burned hairs of the offending dog into the wound. The beard was once considered so important that oaths were uttered over it. In the well-known fairy tale, the three little pigs swore such an oath when they cried, "Not by the hair of my chinny, chin, chin."

A symbol of strength, love, beauty and rank, hair can also be an emblem of evil. Scandinavians once believed eyebrows that met above the nose were the sign of a witch, wizard or werewolf. Werewolves, werefoxes and other hairy creatures are symbols of the beast in man in almost every culture. Satan and his demonic hordes are often portrayed bristling with hair. In the Middle Ages, fat from the body of a dead red-haired person was used as an ingredient in poisons.

Part of hair's magic, the reason it is such a ready and powerful symbol, lies in its versatility. Although hair is a part of the body, it can be cut without bleeding or pain, sacrificed and preserved, shorn and regrown. Hair yields to braiding, dyeing, bleaching, frizzing and curling. In decorating the body, hair is the most obvious place to start.

The early Egyptians, four millennia before the birth of Christ, wore their own hair. But by 2000 B.C., Egypt's upper classes were shaving their heads and wearing wigs. Reflecting the rank of the wearer, most wigs were elaborate adornments, never intended to look like real hair.

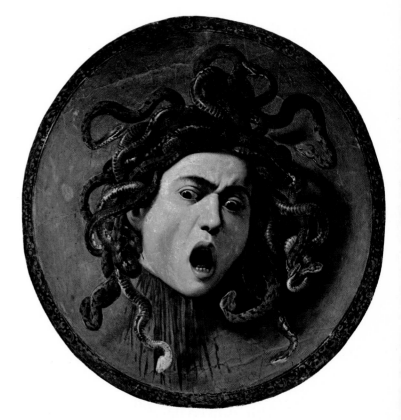

The Greek maiden Medusa paid a terrible price for her alluring hair. Its beauty attracted the ocean god Poseidon, and she foolishly yielded to his advances in the temple of Athena, virgin goddess of wisdom. Outraged at the sacrilege, Athena transformed Medusa's hair into a nest of serpents. Thereafter, one look at her horrible countenance turned a man to stone.

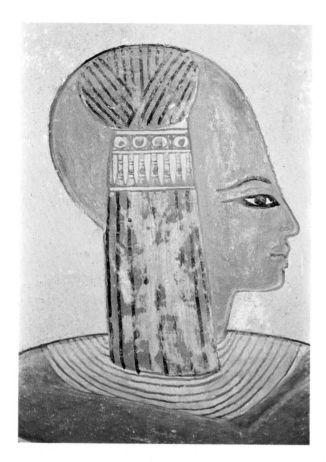

Members of ancient Egypt's upper classes began shaving their heads and wearing elaborate wigs around 2000 B.C. Young boys kept one long lock of twisted or braided hair, which was sometimes dyed and usually worn over the right shoulder.

Black was the favored color, but by 1200 B.C., red, blue and green were also fashionable. Young boys kept one long lock of hair on their shaved heads, usually on the right side. Beards also symbolized social worth in ancient Egypt. Pharaohs and their queens both wore false beards, sometimes hair powdered with gold, sometimes threads of gold or other metals.

Around the Mediterranean, long hair and beards were common, although styles varied from place to place. Ancient Persians considered the shaven face an absurdity. But the Hittites shaved beard, mustache, eyebrows and even a patch of hair at the temple. Around 1700 B.C., Cretan men sported a roach, a bristly band of hair running front to back across a shaven head. This style was briefly revived in America in the 1950s and 1960s, when it was called the Mohawk. Barbarians shaved their beards but not their mustaches. Richard Corson, a historian of hair, has written that the fashion "offended both the bearded and the shaven peoples exceedingly."

The most powerful of the Greek gods, Zeus and Poseidon, displayed full beards and long hair. Greeks wore their hair long until about the sixth century B.C. Hair styles of men and women were similar. Beards endured until the fourth century B.C., when Alexander the Great ordered his soldiers to shave so that Persian soldiers would have no convenient handles with which to grab Greek heads.

Early Romans wore beards and combed their short hair forward. In 297 B.C., Sicilian barbers landed in Rome and soon started a fashion of clean-shavenness. Young men consecrated their first beard to the gods. Emperor Nero, never one for half measures, preserved his imperial peach fuzz in a golden box encrusted with pearls. Some Roman men wore wigs to hide their baldness. Others painted their heads. The Roman senate granted Julius Caesar the privilege of wearing his laurel wreath whenever he chose, a gift of great importance to a vain and balding dictator.

Around the time of the birth of Christ, Roman law required prostitutes to wear blond wigs as a sign of their profession. Messalina, third wife of the emperor Claudius I, singlehandedly dismantled the law by wearing a yellow wig on her

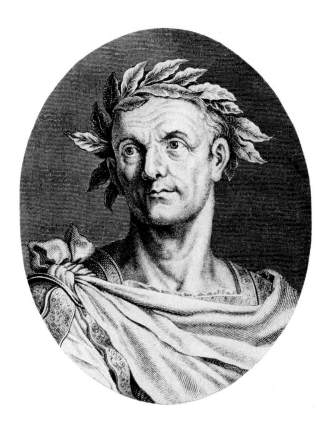

Of all the tributes rendered unto Julius Caesar, permission from the Roman senate to wear his laurel wreath at all times was among those of which he was proudest. Caesar's embarrassment over his baldness indirectly influenced the historical standard for royal headgear. His wreath supposedly served as the original model for the more elaborate golden crowns of European monarchs in later centuries.

nighttime tours through the seedier districts of the city. When the regulation was lifted, yellow wigs became so popular that the Roman satirist Martial quipped:

> The golden hair that Galla wears
> Is hers — who would have thought it?
> She swears 'tis hers, and true she swears,
> For I know where she bought it.

Perfumes, oils, colors and other decorations of the hair were common with the Romans. One observer noted that Commodus, emperor between 180 and 192 A.D., had hair that "glittered from its natural whiteness, and from the quantity of essences and gold dust with which it was loaded, so that when the sun was shining, it might have been thought that his head was on fire." When the Romans conquered Gaul and Britain, they found barbarians with hair dyed red, green, orange and blue.

By the end of the second century, the early fathers of the Christian Church had begun to rail against the current fashions, a practice that has continued for centuries. Clement of Alexandria cautioned his flock that priestly benedictions bestowed at worship services could not penetrate wigs. One could have false hair or grace, but not both. His contemporary, Tertullian, warned that "the fake hair you wear may have come not only from a criminal but from a very dirty head, perhaps from the head of one already damned."

Charlemagne sported a beard and long hair as he bent much of Europe to his will, but when he became Holy Roman Emperor, he adopted the Church's dictates and commanded his subjects to shave. In the eighth century, a haircut was still an important event. A young male child's first haircut was usually performed by a respected friend or relative who thereafter acted as godfather to the boy.

In the Middle Ages, the Church succeeded, to some extent, in regulating hair fashions. But settling on an acceptable style was no simple matter, even for churchmen. Monks' tonsures varied from country to country and no predominant style was ever agreed upon. Scotch Catholics preferred a semicircular tonsure, a horseshoe of hair around the head, called the tonsure of St. John.

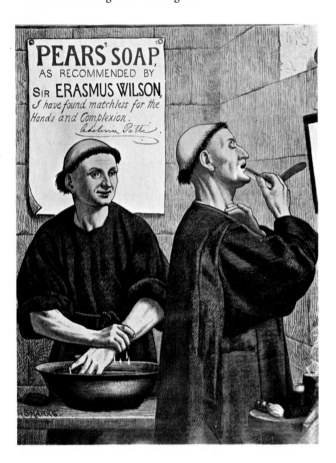

The tonsure of St. Peter, a circular tonsure like a halo of hair, was the favored style in Germany, Spain and Italy. Britain's St. Wulstan, Bishop of Worcester, pronounced long hair "highly immoral, criminal and beastly." A man of action, he carried a knife up his sleeve and lopped off a hank of hair from any shaggy penitent who knelt to receive his blessing. Some Crusaders, imitating their Saracen foes, returned from the East with illicit beards. The growing popularity of facial hair prompted the Archbishop of Rouen to warn in 1096 that men with beards were in danger of damnation. In 1105, Bishop Serlo persuaded England's King Henry I to submit to a trim and a shave and produced a pair of scissors on the spot. Henry's court followed suit, eclipsing beards as a fashion in England.

Monks and priests were the physicians and surgeons of the Middle Ages, at least until 1163. In that year the Council of Tours forbade men of the cloth to practice surgery. Their assistants, the barbers, quickly assumed the responsibility. The first barber's guild, The Worshipful Company of Barbers, was formed in England in 1308. Some specialization took place, and until the middle of the eighteenth century, barbers and surgeons quarreled over exactly who was fit to apply the blade to what part of the body. The surgeons eventually formed their own guild in 1745.

Although the Church enforced its opinions with a heavy hand, the Middle Ages were not without fashion and vanity. When women uncovered their heads in about the thirteenth century, they arranged their hair in great looping braids that arched out over their ears. Dye, ribbons, wool and false hair added to the hair styles. During this period, European women first plucked their eyebrows and scalp to refine their appearance, a common practice ever since. Blond hair was especially popular. Some women dyed their hair blond, or wore wigs. Others sat in the moonlight hoping to capture a mysterious glow that they believed would give them blond hair.

In fourteenth-century Spain, men wore beards of different colors and styles for different occasions. The ease with which gentlemen could disguise themselves sometimes led to shenanigans, causing Peter, King of Aragon, to outlaw false beards. In the fifteenth century, older men began to exhibit beards as a sign of rank and prestige. English law, however, decreed that "no manner of man that will be taken for an Englishman shall have no beard above his mouth."

The King's Burnt Hair

After men had worn their hair long for a hundred years, the misfortune of a king prompted a turnabout in men's hair styles. In 1521, Francis I of France, out for an evening's fun, rounded up his companions and with a great flurry of snowballs stormed the house of his friend Count Montgomery. Carrying the defense too far, one of the Count's guests or servants flung a torch at the invaders, singeing the king's hair. On his doctor's orders, Francis cut his hair. To stay in step with the monarch, French dandies followed the fashion. England's King Henry VIII admired the new style and copied it. In 1535, the king

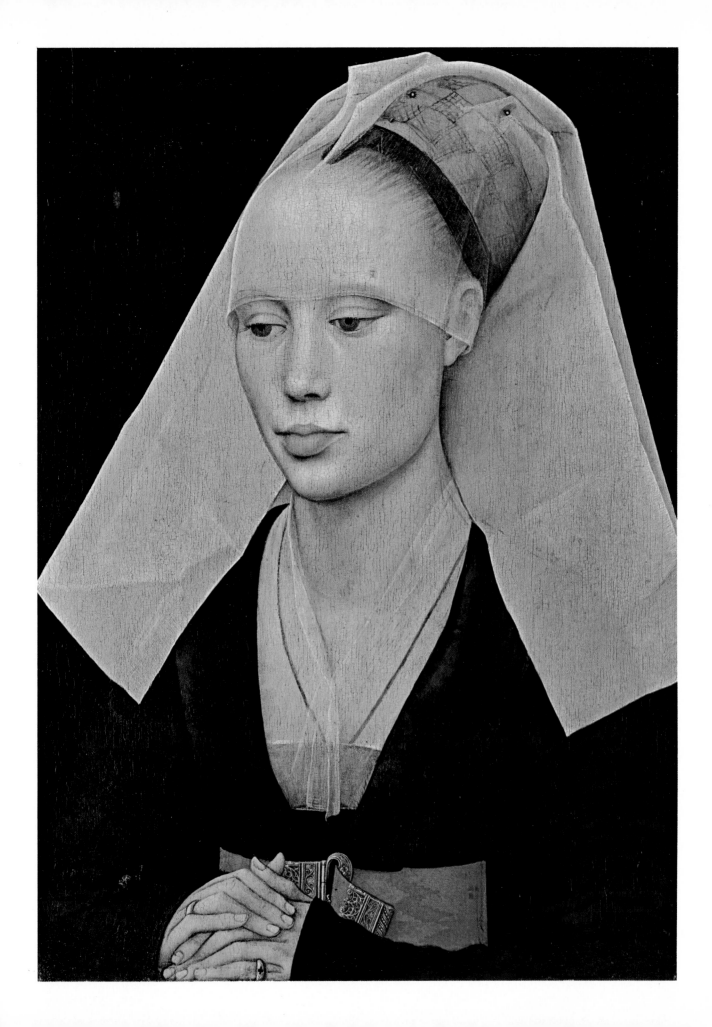

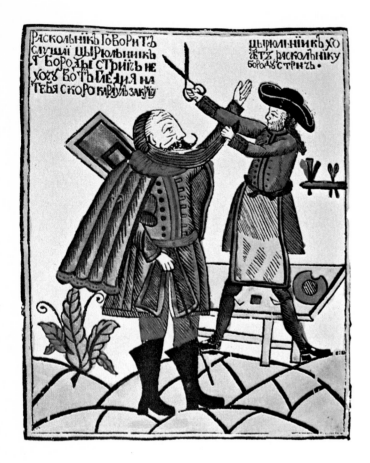

In 1698, Russia's Peter the Great imposed a tax on beards. Local collectors enforced the law at city gates. Bearded men who refused to pay were often relieved of their whiskers by force.

"commanded all about his Court to poll their heads, and to give them example, he caused his own head to be polled." The influence of the kings lasted until the end of the century.

Beards flourished in the sixteenth century as never before. "Men usually like to have a reasonable display of hair somewhere on the head," writes Corson. "It may be the hair or it may be the beard. They seldom want both long hair and long beards at the same time, and they are rarely contented for very long with short hair and no beards. Therefore, when the hair came off, the beards were allowed to grow. Henry encouraged this and set no limits on size or style." Beards were waxed, dyed, powdered and perfumed. Styles included French, Spanish, Dutch, Italian, old, new, mean, common, court, spade, fantail, forked, bush and sugar-loaf. The prodigious beard of Hans Steiniger, the burgermeister of Brannau, Austria, ended his political career and his life. Herr Steiniger normally tucked his eight-foot, nine-inch-long beard into his garments to ascend the stairs to the council chambers. But on September 28, 1567, he forgot. On the way up, he tripped over his beard and bounced back down the stairs to his doom.

Throughout the 1500s, most women parted their hair in the middle, tied it back or braided it. Many married women kept their hair covered, revealing it to no one but their husbands. By the end of the sixteenth century, wigs had become popular. It was during this time that the term periwig — since shortened to wig — came into use. Queen Elizabeth I had many wigs, usually fashioned in tight red or yellow curls. English women dyed, curled or frizzed their hair in imitation of hers.

In the seventeenth century, a monarch's whim again set the fashion for hair. Louis XIII, blessed with abundant hair in his youth, began to grow bald with age. He put on a wig in 1624, and soon all of France wore false hair. Louis XIV, France's Sun King, suffered from the same pilar dwindling and set a huge cascading wig on his head at age thirty-five. During his lifetime, it is said, no one but his barber, Binette, saw Louis XIV without a wig. Fashionable men wore wigs for more than a century, and one wit offered an instructive example to all men who chose to cloak their heads in someone else's ageless hair:

His hair will never know a fall,
'Tis ever dark and curly;
Be wise if you wear wigs at all
Like him adopt one early.

The rise of the wig sent beards into decline. By the end of the century, they vanished altogether under the razor. Even when retained, the very names of seventeenth-century beards suggested their diminutive size: the needle, the stiletto and the Roman T. In 1698, Peter the Great tried to eradicate the beard in Russia with a beard tax. Tax collectors at the gates of Russian towns stopped nobleman and peasant alike. A wealthy man might pay roughly $45 to keep his beard. The beard tax for peasants was about three cents.

As in our own times, fashions were sometimes strenuously resisted. When England was split by civil war, Puritans purposely turned away from the elaborate wigs of the king's Cavaliers and adopted a simple bowl cut that earned them the name Roundheads. In 1653, pastor Thomas Hall published *The Loathesomeness of Long Haire,* in which he confidently asserted that "where one wicked man wear short hair, there is a thousand weare long." In America, Harvard University forbade long hair in 1655. Another fashion, a single braid of hair hanging over one shoulder, the lovelock, provoked considerable indignation. In England, William Prynne spoke out against the new style with his scathing *The Unloveliness, of Love-lockes, or A summary Discourse, proving: The wearing, and nourishing of a Locke, or Love-Locke, to be altogether unseemly, and unlawful unto Christians.*

Women's coiffures, tall at the beginning of the seventeenth century, grew even taller by the end. Every curl and lock had a name. Confidants were small curls near the ears. Creve-coeurs, or heart-breakers, were curls hanging at the nape of the neck. Locks dangling at the temples were called favorites. Women piled their own hair, and hair borrowed from other heads, on wire frames called commodes. Pads, oils and a shiny grease known as pomade or pomatum were needed to keep the elaborate styles in place. One popular style, the fontange, first appeared by accident.

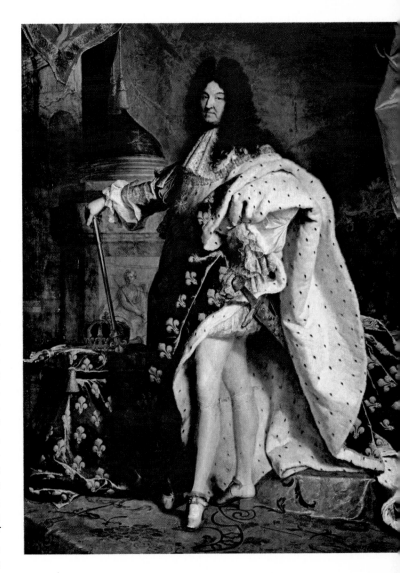

Louis XIV of France reportedly employed forty wig makers to keep himself fashionably coiffed. Vanity came easily to heads of state. No one but the king's personal barber, Binette, was allowed to see Louis without a wig.

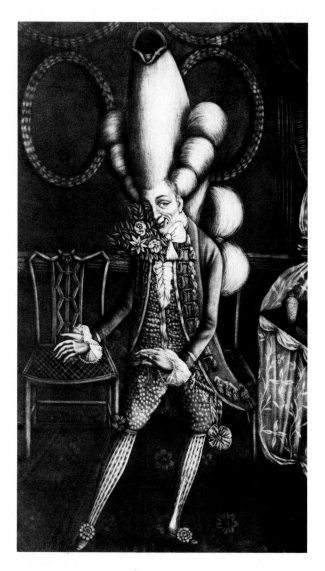

A tower of false hair stretched over a wire frame, elaborate side curls and a long queue, doubled over itself to form the "club," were the distinctive features of the Macaroni hair style. The Macaronis, subjects of many caricatures, were a group of rich, idle English fops who traveled through Italy on a grand tour in the 1770s. They returned to England to found the Macaroni club, parade their new coiffures and irritate many of their countrymen.

While riding with King Louis XIV of France, the Duchesse de Fontanges, his mistress, had the misfortune to have her coiffure fall apart. She tied her hair up with her garter, an improvisation that delighted the king. Soon, the most fashionable women of France were wearing tousled towers of hair laced with ribbons, in imitation of the duchess's impromptu hairdo.

With the success of Legros de Rumigny, a cook who traded in his spoon for a comb, Paris became the center of hairdressing. By 1769, the city had 1,200 hairdressers. Competition soon drove coiffures literally through the roof. "Women's styles," says Corson, "move in a clearly defined pattern from a peak of artificiality at the end of the seventeenth century through a disarming trough of simplicity in the first half of the eighteenth, rising at last to a crescendo of excess which could scarcely have been imagined, let alone anticipated, a few years before." Women of fashion sometimes had to kneel in carriages to fit both themselves and their hair inside. Doorways became higher as a result of the fashion. One inventive hair stylist created a mechanical hairdo that could be lowered a foot or two by pressing a spring. Unable to fit in a carriage on her way to a ball, Marie Antoinette chose a convertible hair style. It apparently rode beside her in the coach and atop her at the ball. Coiffures had a variety of unusual names, such as the Chest of Drawers, the Mad Dog and the Drowned Chicken. Huge ostrich feathers, a favorite of Marie Antoinette, were popular. Elaborate artifices depicted allegorical tales, scenes from plays, poems, gardens, Parisian buildings and even hot-air balloons.

The sticky pomades needed to hold all this hair, real and false, on elaborate scaffolding often gave high fashion a bad smell. Beef marrow was a common ingredient. One ode to fashion in a newspaper of the period warned women:

> When he scents the mingled steam
> Which your plaster'd heads are rich in,
> Lard and meal, and clouted cream,
> Can he love a walking kitchen?

When Marie Antoinette bore a child, she temporarily lost much of her hair, so short hair became the fashion. By the turn of the century,

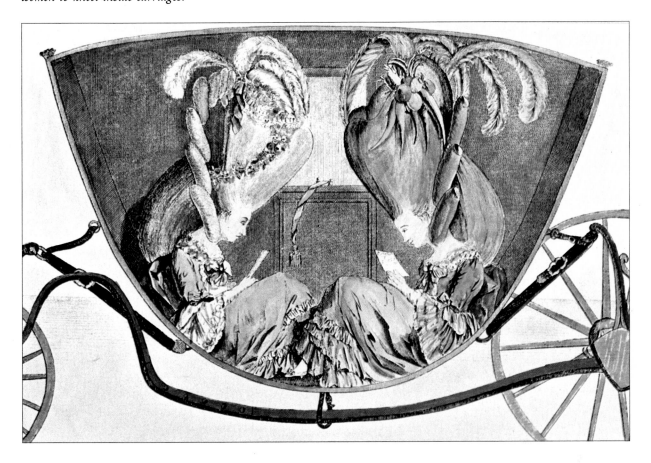

curls had replaced the towering constructions of earlier decades. The French Revolution, in its repudiation of the excesses of the *ancien régime,* ushered in shorter styles. Some featured a row of curls above an exposed neck, as if mockingly inviting the guillotine. One such style was called *la coiffure à la victime.* Late in the eighteenth century and through much of the nineteenth, women made jewelry, portraits and pictures out of clippings from their hair. Some families wove strands from every member into a floral design, a kind of family flower.

For men, the eighteenth century was the age of the wig. As wigs grew smaller at the beginning of the 1700s, they became less expensive, and more people adopted them. Men who could not afford wigs imitated them with their own hair. A great part of this deception was powdering. Every fashionable house had a powder room. To trap the powder, wigs were greased slightly. The face was masked and the clothes covered with a cloak as a servant powdered the hairpiece. Wheat flour was preferred, but riots early in the century over wasting the nutritious powder on gentlemen's hair started a search for alternatives.

Wigs of the period either simply covered the head or had long queues stretching down the back. Soldiers sometimes protected their clothes by tying their queues in bags, which began a vogue for the bag-wig. Certain wig styles became professional badges. With so many men wearing wigs, self-consciousness about false hair was not a problem. Feeling a draft at a public ceremony in Poland, Peter the Great reached down, plucked the wig from the crown of a nearby gentleman and dropped it on his own head.

In the 1770s, a group of young London fops returning from Italy formed the Macaroni Club and flaunted their own remarkable hair style, the Macaroni. It featured a wall of hair rising straight up from the forehead, huge curls on either side and a long queue doubled over itself in a style called the club. Londoners almost instantly began to ridicule the new hair style. One verse of a popular song, *The Macaroni,* sneered:

This fashion who does e'er pursue,
I think a simple-tony;
For he's a fool, say what you will,
Who is a Macaroni.

The term Macaroni eventually came to mean any outrageous fashion, not just a ridiculous hairdo. This use of the word found a place in American popular song when Yankee Doodle stuck a feather in his cap and called it "Macaroni."

In an age when almost everyone wore wigs, fashionable folk sometimes fell victim to a crime unknown to other times — wig-naping. Well-dressed Londoners occasionally had their hair snatched off their heads in broad daylight. Some thieves yanked the wig off a victim's head and threw it to a dog that was trained to dash off with it. At least one man lost his hairpiece when a thief cut through the back of his coach and spirited the wig away.

Gradually, the popularity of wigs began to wane. Their association with royalty and aristocracy lent them an air of privilege in an age of revolution and democracy. Britain imposed a tax on powder for wigs in 1795, which brought in 200,000 pounds in its first year. As the popularity of wigs declined, so did the revenues. In America, beards and mustaches had long since fallen from favor, perhaps as a result of the plain styles of living advocated by the Puritans. Although a few patriots still wore wigs, not one signer of the Declaration of Independence sported facial hair of any kind. By the early nineteenth century, wigs had all but disappeared.

For women, small topknots sometimes flanked by braids or curls around the ears were fashionable in the early decades of the nineteenth century. Many young women wore flowers in their hair. By the middle of the century, the chignon, a large, round roll or knot of hair at the back of the head or neck, ruled the world of fashion. Because the chignon demanded more hair than most women had, it prompted a return to long hair,

sometimes several feet of it, and brought false hair, but not wigs, back into favor.

By the 1860s, the chignon had spawned a generation of smaller curls and buns to adorn the head. "Perfect scaffoldings of hair are now built upon the head," said *Godey's Lady's Book* magazine, "roll upon roll — puff upon puff." One extraordinary style of the period demanded "two rats, two mice, a cat and a cataract." A reader hardy enough to continue reading the article learned that "the rats are the long frizzets of curled hair for the side rolls; the mice are the smaller ones above them; the cat is [the name] for the roll laid over the top of the head; and the cataract is for the chignon at the back of the head — which is sometimes called waterfall, cataract, and *jet d'eau.*" The chignon was the subject of some particularly ungentlemanly abuse. "This tumor-like excrescence," a writer bellowed in the *Bazar Book of Decorum,* "disfigures the top of the head with the appearance of a horrid growth of disease which would seem to call for the knife of a surgeon did we not know that it could be placed or displaced at the will of the wearer." Outbursts of this kind had as little effect on fashion then as they have now. Women continued to wear their hair as they pleased.

The chignon helped make hair merchants a common sight in Europe, especially in France and Germany. Poor peasant girls lined up to be shorn, parting with their long tresses for trinkets, clothes or a few coins. Hair was also shorn from corpses and prisoners. In 1859-60, almost 200,000 pounds of hair valued at more than $1 million was shipped to America from Europe. The hair trade tripled by 1866.

Curls, fringes, frizzes and waves began to take precedence over the chignon in the late nineteenth century. In the 1870s, a French stablehand turned hairdresser, Marcel Grateau, invented a process for waving hair that was adopted almost universally over the next fifty years. By turning a curling iron upside down, he could put a soft, lasting wave in hair rather than a tight curl. His creation, the marcel wave, grew so popular that Grateau's customers competed for his services. The highest bidder won a head rippling with marcels from the hands of the master himself. He retired at the age of forty-five, rich, famous and, by all accounts, happy.

Short, curly hair combed forward was the most popular style for men early in the nineteenth century. Whiskers, although not full beards, also enjoyed renewed prominence. Oils and greases to shine and control hair became popular. The finest concoction of the day, Macassar oil, was even praised by the poet Lord Byron:

> In virtues nothing earthly could surpass her,
> Save thine 'incomparable oil,' Macassar!

So many men took to wearing hair salves that women were driven to protect the backs and arms of their furniture with pieces of lace or cloth known as antimacassars. Byron's hair style, curly and slightly longer than most, was a particular favorite of dandies of his time. Other fops imitated Beau Brummell, a London fashion plate who reportedly required three hairdressers to tend to his pampered hair — one for the side curls, one for the front and one for the back.

Jailed for a Beard

Outlandish hairdos often brought mockery, but not violence. Beards, for the first half of the nineteenth century, were another matter. When a forty-two-year-old butcher and farmer, Joseph Palmer, moved to Fitchburg, Massachusetts in 1830, men jeered at him, women crossed the street to avoid passing near him and children pelted him with rocks and stones, all because Palmer wore a long, full beard.

A veteran of the War of 1812, a friend of Ralph Waldo Emerson and Henry David Thoreau, Palmer ignored his community's abuses as long as he could. But one Sunday, denied communion in the local church, Palmer rose to his feet, walked to the communion table and raised the cup to his lips, saying, "I am a better Christian than any of you." Soon after, Palmer was attacked in the street by four men and thrown to the ground. One of the men pulled out a pair of scissors and tried to trim Palmer's beard, but Palmer drew a pocketknife from his trousers and slashed two of the men in the legs, driving them off. The local constable arrested him for "unprovoked assault." When Palmer refused to pay a

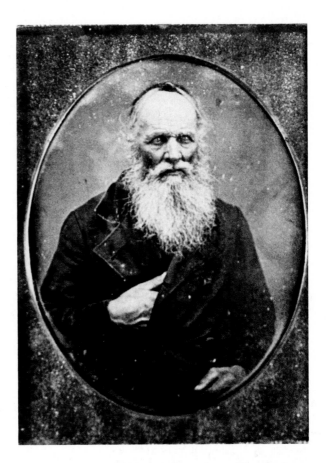

Joseph Palmer glares defiantly from behind the beard that men jeered at and women crossed the street to avoid. In 1830, a few citizens of Palmer's town, clean-shaven Fitchburg, Massachusetts, were so offended by his beard that they attacked him in the street and tried to cut it off. Refusing to pay a fine for this public offense, Palmer was judged the guilty party in the assault and sentenced to a year in jail.

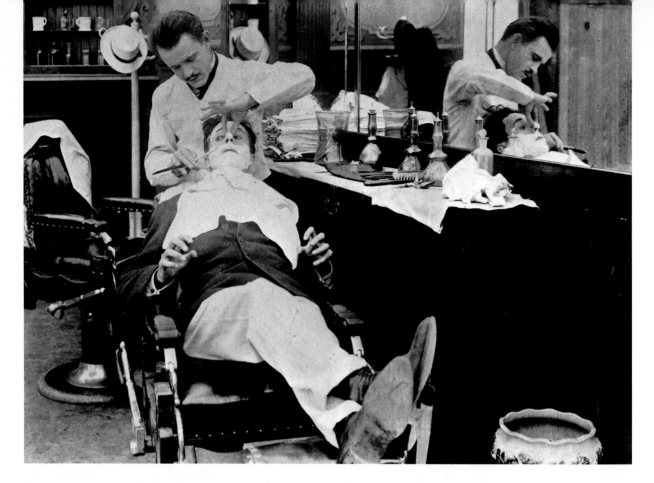

The hydraulic barber chair made shaving more comfortable for everyone. Of course, the barber's skill might still leave room for terror, as this scene from the 1915 comedy Beppo the Barber *illustrates.*

fine, he was sentenced to jail. His jailers kept Palmer in solitary confinement for much of his year in prison. Five men once tried to cut off his beard, but he thrashed two of them and chased the others off. By smuggling out letters through his son, Palmer eventually attracted the attention of local newspapers. He became such an embarrassment to officials that, near the end of his term, they opened his cell and told him he could go free. "You put me in here," Palmer responded, "and you'll have to put me out." Hoisting him into a chair, they carried him outside and set him down on the sidewalk. Palmer lived in Fitchburg for another forty years. His gravestone, decorated with a likeness of his bearded face, bears the words, "Persecuted for wearing the beard."

By the second half of the century, beards, mustaches and side whiskers were commonplace, if not universal. The fashion did not flourish unchallenged, however. In 1850, the *Knickerbocker* magazine declared that "every principle of comity and social order" cried out for the abolition of beards. "There exists no right whatever," the article went on, "to exhibit to the community . . . a disgusting object of this sort." The whiskers of General Ambrose Burnside earned his name, more or less, a place in history — sideburns. Long

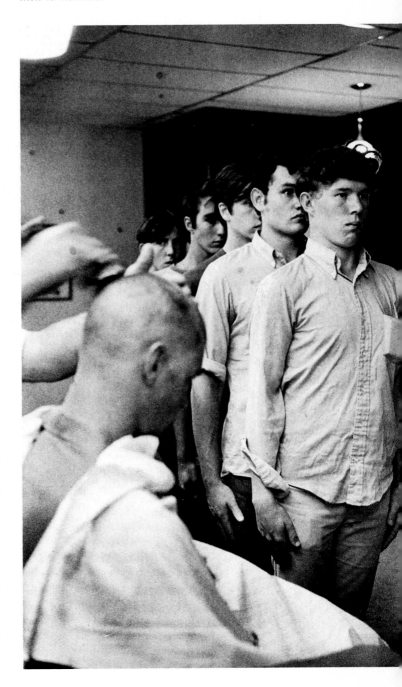

For much of the twentieth century, boot camp was the hub of fashion for men's hair styles. Two world wars put millions of men in uniform and brought the crew cut to soldiers and then to civilians.

whiskers hanging several inches from the jowls were known as Piccadilly Weepers. Particularly extreme weepers bore the name Dundrearies, after the impressive growth on the cheeks of Lord Dundreary, a character in English playwright Tom Taylor's play, *Our American Cousin*. By the 1860s, even our American president, Abraham Lincoln, sported a beard. Lincoln spent the last moments of his life at Ford's Theater watching *Our American Cousin*, perhaps amused at Lord Dundreary's Dundrearies. Eight of the next ten presidents wore beards or mustaches.

The last decade of the nineteenth century brought forth two innovations that revolutionized barbering. The first was the hydraulic barber's chair, which allowed men to lean back in comfort as their barbers raised and lowered them to the perfect height. But much more important was the disposable razor blade, developed by American inventor King Camp Gillette in 1895. In 1903, he sold 51 razors and 168 blades. The next year he sold 90,000 razors and 12 million blades. Hydraulic chairs notwithstanding, men began to shave at home.

The Constancy of Change

Men's hair styles remained uniformly short from the beginning of the twentieth century until the mid-1950s. The military haircut of World War I became, with only a few variations, the crew cut of mid-century. Beards and mustaches did not survive long into this century. "A German scientist estimates," one polemicist wrote, "that 2,000,000 misanthropic microbes can find accommodation in 'an average beard. . . . ' It is no pleasing thing to feel that when one is talking to a bearded man one is in the presence of a huge invisible army which may at any moment send forth a brigade, a battalion, a sergeant or two, intent upon the invasion of one's self." A French scientist sent two men — one bearded, one clean-shaven — through the streets of Paris for a few hours and then had each, in turn, kiss his assistant. When he brushed her lips and deposited the invisible remnants of the clean-shaven man's kiss in a laboratory dish, he found only harmless yeasts and a few other hitchhikers. The kiss of the bearded man carried the hair of a spider's leg,

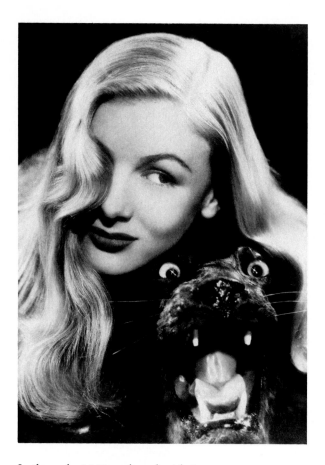

In the early 1940s, when short hair had dominated women's fashion for twenty years, Veronica Lake single-handedly began a temporary return to longer hair. She first displayed her seductive hair style in the movie I Wanted Wings *in 1941.*

tubercule bacilli and other alarming particles. Science, summoned to fashion's defense, helped dictate beardlessness for the next fifty years.

In the first two decades of the twentieth century, women wore elaborate hair styles piled high with curls, buns and deep waves. Wigs came back into fashion. A German-born hairdresser working in London, Karl Nessler, capitalized on the bold coiffures of the period. He invented the first machine for sculpting permanent waves into hair, the precursor of modern permanents. Under the name of Charles Nestlé, he moved his business from London to New York, where his procedure won him wealth and fame. One of Nestlé's early permanents took up to twelve hours to complete and could cost $1,000.

World War I dealt a blow to this kind of intricate fashion. In France, Britain and America, the war drove women into industry and made a hazard of their long hair. The boldest women cut their hair short. By the mid-1920s the shorter styles had become fashionable. Dancer Irene Castle brought her bobbed hair from Paris to London to the United States. She may have been responsible for more shearing than any other person in history. American women strode into barber shops by the thousands to cast off their long hair. Matrons, men and moralists raged against the new fashion. "A 'bobbed' woman," one preacher howled, "is a disgraced woman! Surely a very serious consideration for all who fear God! What will the Lord say to our sisters about this when we all stand at His judgment seat?" The cries of convention had no effect. Variations on the bob abounded, with names like the Chesterfield, the Horseshoe, the Gigolo and the Coconut. When film stars Clara Bow and Mary Pickford bobbed their hair, they reinforced the trend.

Another movie star, Veronica Lake, briefly overwhelmed the bob with a long, wavy, seductive mane of blond hair that hung sleepily over one eye. Called the bad-girl style, Lake's locks alarmed moralists even more than the bob. But the style did not last long, perhaps because of the peril of navigating one-eyed through life. *Life* magazine also noted that Miss Lake's hair "catches fire fairly often when she is smoking."

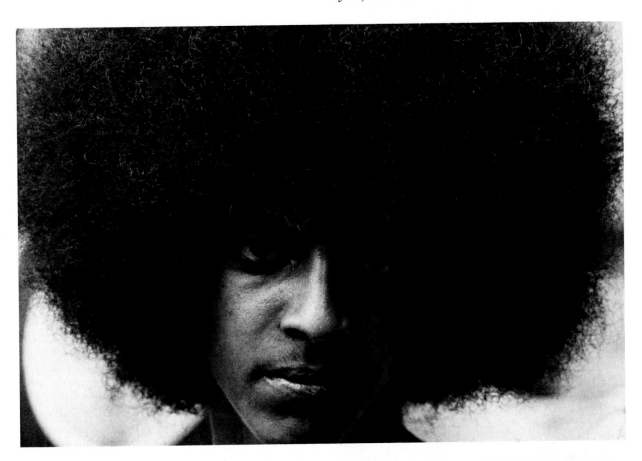

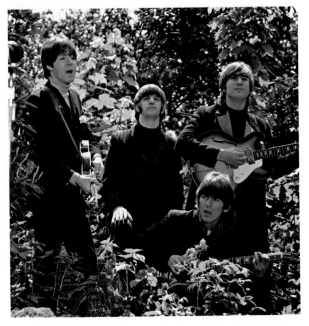

The early 1950s saw some women cutting their hair almost to the scalp, in imitation of the crew cut. Anticipating a common complaint of a later era, but from the opposite point of view, writer Robert Ruark quipped, "You have to ask for a draft card to tell boys from girls."

In the late 1950s, hair styles of both men and women began to vary with an inventiveness that has persisted to this day. Bouffants and beehives brought business and renewed respect to hairdressers and wigmakers. Home permanents and hair dryers let nearly every woman try her hand at new styles. Between 1960 and 1970, total sales of false hair in America increased from $4 million to $500 million.

The crew cut met its match in Elvis Presley and the Beatles. Presley's long, slicked-back hair topped with a few wild black locks drooping over his forehead began a return to longer hair for men in the late 1950s. His induction into the

From crew cut to uncut, hair styles
evolved through the 1950s and
1960s. Part of hair's usefulness as a
symbol lies in its versatility. In
every age and culture, hair expresses
some part of the person beneath it.

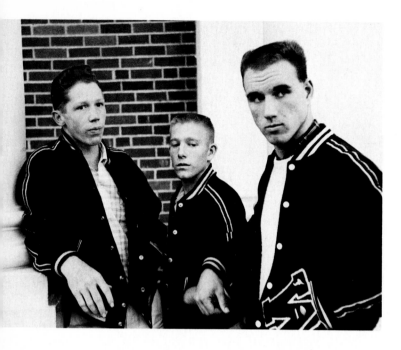

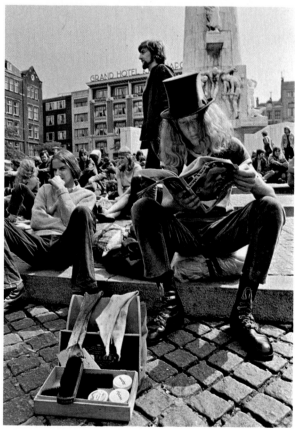

army slowed the change of fashion temporarily, but the arrival of the Beatles in the United States in 1964 caused hair to sprout everywhere. The early hair styles of the Beatles, which hid only their foreheads and the tops of their collars and ears, now seem tame. But high schools across the United States refused to give diplomas to long-haired seniors. Some principals took matters into their own hands by shearing students on the spot, just as Britain's Bishop of Worcester had forcibly sheared his flock centuries before. In 1968, the citizens of Norwalk, Connecticut paid for a billboard near the train station that showed a long-haired teen-ager surrounded by the words, "Students of Norwalk, Beautify America, Get a Haircut." More than one school district found itself in court defending its right to ban long hair on boys. Opposition to long hair occasionally grew violent. On May 7, 1970, a fifteen-year-old California boy was admitted to a hospital after two men tried to scalp him because they considered his long hair un-American.

Young women began wearing their hair long and straight and ironed it regularly to keep it that way. Blacks adopted the Afro and met the same kind of resistance encountered by men who grew their hair long. One airline fired a stewardess for wearing an Afro aloft. American hair styles were adopted abroad. In Mexico, Brazil and Argentina, men with long hair were arrested and trimmed. Czechoslovakia and Bulgaria stopped long-haired men at their borders. Singapore, Indonesia, South Vietnam and Thailand had restrictions on the length of hair.

During the 1970s, long hair on young men attained a kind of acceptability. High school students were often permitted to wear their hair as they wished. Older men began sporting longer sideburns, mustaches, beards and hair that crept over their ears. The armed forces grudgingly accepted short, neat beards and mustaches on servicemen. But the incorporation of long hair into respectable fashion did not end the usefulness of hair styles as a form of protest.

In England, from the mid-1960s to the present, a succession of youth cults have adopted extreme hair styles and fashions. The mods of the 1960s, who wore their hair short and neat, struggled,

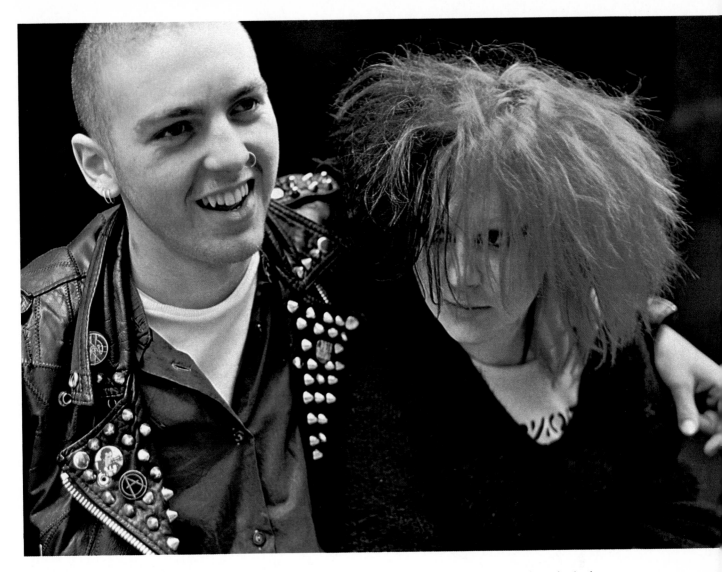

sometimes violently, with the slick-haired rockers, who idolized Elvis Presley and the young Marlon Brando. The skinheads of the early 1970s supplanted both in notoriety by shaving their heads to the scalp and loudly proclaiming their disaffection with nearly everyone: mods, rockers, hippies, squares and especially foreigners. Punks combined wild hair styles in vivid colors with the anger and alienation of the skinheads.

Only the variety of hair styles remains constant. In any culture, hair is perhaps the most versatile medium of physical self-expression. Holding enduring associations with sexuality, strength, good and evil, hair's symbolic variations are inexhaustible and powerful. In every century and culture, a simple change in hair style has the power to provoke responses varying from outrage to admiration. It always speaks of the individual it adorns, through its simplicity or elaborateness, its neglect or artistry.

The late 1970s brought forth a new fashion in music, dress, hair styles and skin-piercing body decoration — punk. From hair at its shortest to hair at its wildest, two British punks capture the outrageous extremes of the tonsorial art.

109

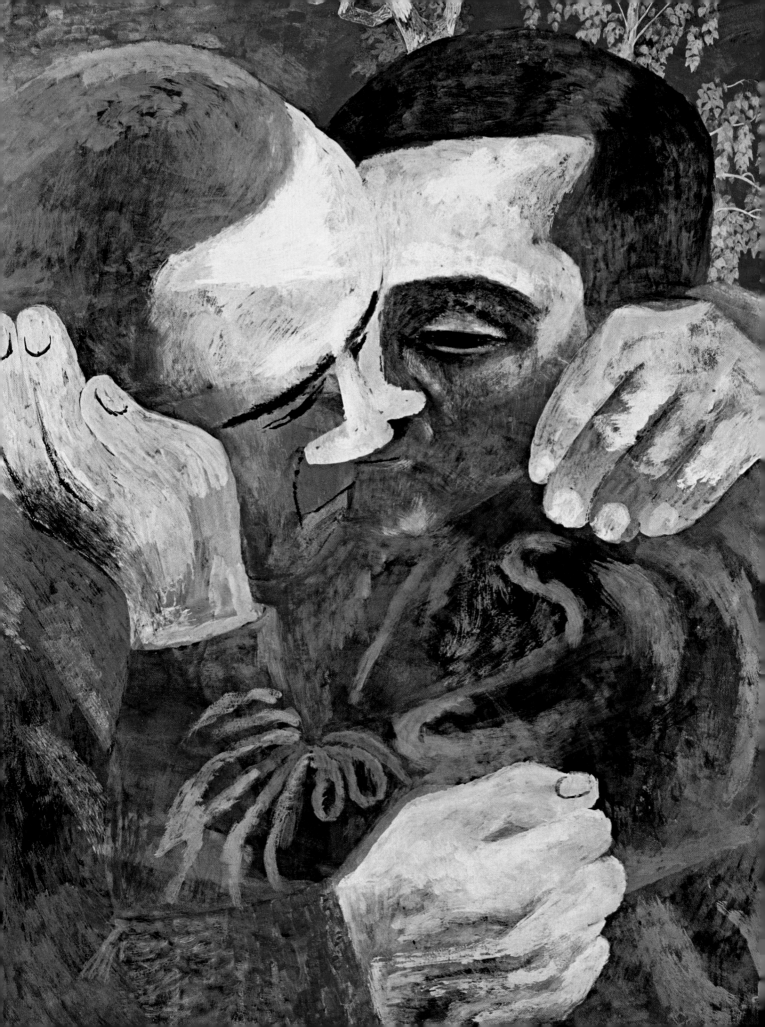

Chapter 5

The Human Touch

"Maybe you're in a wheelchair or on crutches," declares television evangelist Ernest Angley, as he extends his outstretched fingers toward the eye of the camera. "Maybe you have a crippled child or a retarded child. Bring it and press it against my hand at the point of contact." His face is contorted by intense concentration. Softly, he intones, "Heal, heal, heal, in the name of the Lord." Gazing into the camera again, he asks, "Don't you feel Him? He's there, making you well. Making your child well." Such is Angley's popularity that each weekend his unique brand of healing airs in nearly every major American city. Millions have heard him and believe that miracles flow from his touch.

The resurgence of faith healing in America stems from the rising tide of fundamentalist Christianity. Faith healers draw their inspiration from the New Testament, in which the apostles recount the miracle healing performed by Jesus. According to St. Matthew, Jesus healed Peter's mother-in-law when she was sick with a fever by simply touching her hand. And according to St. Luke, "Now when the sun was setting all they that had any sick with divers diseases brought them unto him; and he laid his hands on every one of them, and healed them. And devils also came out of many, crying out, and saying, Thou art Christ the Son of God."

Controversy has attended faith healing from the beginning. The seventeenth-century Irish healer Valentine Greatrakes was an ordinary country squire until he had "an impulse or a strange persuasion" to begin healing. When Greatrakes failed to cure Viscountess Conway of her blinding migraine headaches, however, he was widely accused of fraud and sparked a national controversy. The father of the modern healing movement in America was Alexander Dowie, a Scottish-born Congregational minister who settled in Chicago in 1893. Although fre-

Arms locked in tender embrace, two brothers cradle each other in this 1946 painting by American artist Ben Shahn. Research has revealed that man's sense of touch is far more complex than previously thought. An array of minute organs in the skin signal heat and cold, pressure and pain. The most fleeting touch, psychologists have discovered, can influence human encounters and profoundly affect our perception of interactions.

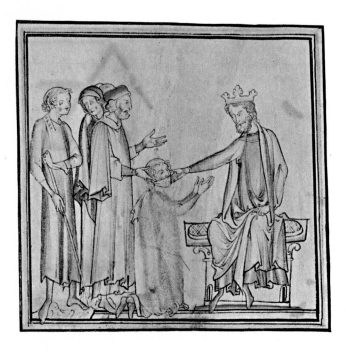

English king Edward the Confessor bestows the Royal Touch on a kneeling subject in a thirteenth-century manuscript. The Royal Touch was thought to cure scrofula, a form of tuberculosis. The custom endured until the early 1700s in England and even longer in France. At his extravagant coronation in 1775, Louis XVI touched 2,400 ailing subjects. He then washed his hands in three napkins, one dipped in vinegar, another in water, the last in perfume.

quently arrested, Dowie attracted thousands of devoted followers with his practice of divine healing. In 1900, he purchased 6,000 acres near Chicago, on which he intended to erect a paradise for the righteous. One year later, he announced that he was "Elijah the Prophet," and eventually his skeptical followers removed him from the head of his own church. By the 1920s, evangelist Aimee Semple McPherson was healing from her California temple. One witness of the healings, writer Carey McWilliams, observed, "When a middle-aged paralytic rose from her wheel chair and took a few stumbling steps, San Diego's legion of incurables, its sick and ailing, started for the platform." McPherson herself later remembered, "Those healings were the topic of conversation on the streets, in hotel lobbies, even in the theatres."

At about the same time, Sinclair Lewis was writing his classic portrait of a philandering religious charlatan, Elmer Gantry. One of Gantry's consorts, the equally guileful Sharon Falconer, ministered healing to a deaf woman. "It amused Sharon," Lewis wrote, "to send out for some oil (it happened to be shotgun oil, but she properly consecrated it) to anoint the woman's ears, and pray lustily for healing."

Despite skeptics, faith healers continue to thrive in America. Once skirting the fringes of established religion, healing has begun moving toward the center. Even the staid Episcopal Church has many members who belong to a healing order, the International Order of St. Luke the Physician. Although healing rests mainly on faith in God, it owes much to the power of touch.

Of all man's senses, touch is dominant. Unlike the others, touch is not localized, like the orbs of delicate tissue that compose the eyes. Touch commands the entire body, from the scalp to the soles of the feet. In a collection of essays, *The World I Live In,* Helen Keller wrote, "Necessity gives to the eye a precious power of seeing, and in the same way it gives a precious power of feeling to the whole body. Sometimes it seems as if the very substance of my flesh were so many eyes looking out at will upon a world newly created every day. . . . It is not for me to say whether we see best with the hand or the eye. I only know that the world I see with my fingers is alive, ruddy, and satisfying. Touch brings the blind many sweet certainties which our more fortunate fellows miss, because their sense of touch is uncultivated." With an unerring touch, blind musicians bring the ring of truth to Keller's words, from jazz pianist George Shearing, to blues and ragtime guitarist Blind Blake, to the incomparable country flatpicker Doc Watson.

Charismatic Christians were not the first to discover the power of touch. The Smith Papyrus, an ancient Egyptian medical text, repeatedly urges physicians to "lay thy hand" upon sores, wounds and ailing parts of the body. In many parts of the world, severed hands and fingers were once supposed to have magical healing properties. Some ancient texts contain accounts of Egyptian women wearing fingers from Jews and Christians for protection against malaria. Later, during the plague years of the Middle Ages, European chiothetists, hand healers, toured the ravaged countryside practicing medicine. In 1423, the English guild of physicians reacted by denouncing "quacks and empirics and knavish men and women." By 1540, England's Parliament had asserted that only men trained at the College of Surgeons were true healers.

A different standard applied to England's kings and queens. For more than 700 years, from the reign of Edward the Confessor until the early eighteenth century, the touch of the English monarch was thought to cure scrofula, a form of tuberculosis. The disease was called the King's Evil. Diarist John Evelyn recorded a ceremony in July 1660, when Charles II bestowed the Royal Touch on a multitude of scrofulous subjects. "His Majesty began to touch for the Evil according to custom, thus: His Majesty sitting under his state in the banqueting house, the chirurgeons cause the sick to be brought, or led, up to the throne, where they kneel; the King strokes their faces or cheeks with both his hands." Among the last people in England to receive the Royal Touch for scrofula was lexicographer Samuel Johnson. In 1712, when he was two years old, Johnson's mother brought him to London for the touch of Queen Anne. His biographer, James Boswell, recorded that when asked if he could remember

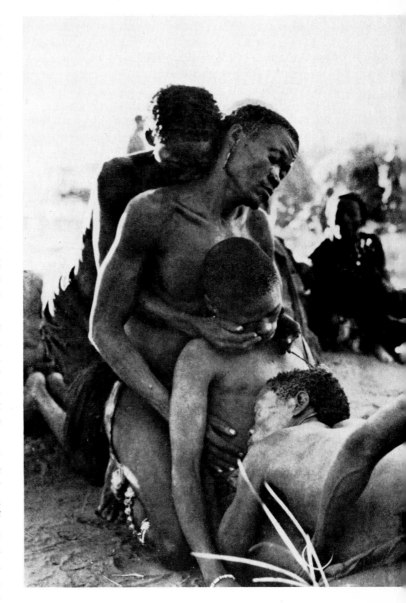

Queen Anne, Johnson replied that he had "a confused, but somehow a sort of solemn recollection of a lady in diamonds, and a long black hood."

Although the bacteria that cause tuberculosis are indifferent to the touch of both king and commoner, the power of touch is indeed formidable. At birth, other senses are limited. While the refinement of sight and hearing takes time, touch remains supreme. In their first weeks of life, babies explore the world through their lips, fingertips and bodies.

Deprivation of Touch

Studies of premature babies have provided insights into the crucial importance of touch. In one study, researchers compared two groups of infants born under normal weight. An experimental group was stroked for five minutes every hour, around the clock, for ten days. The other group, a control group, had routine nursery care. After ten days, the babies who had been handled were gaining weight faster, were more active and appeared to cry less. Perhaps more significant, they were healthier and more active seven to eight months later.

Another study provided dramatic confirmation that touching and stimulation of the skin were critical to premature infants. At one hospital, scientists discovered premature babies gained more weight when their incubators were lined with lamb's wool than when they rested on ordinary cotton sheets. One investigator of this phenomenon, psychologist Martin Richards of Cambridge University, wondered whether the babies were moving less and therefore conserving energy, or whether the lamb's wool was a good insulator, cutting heat loss. Even if both assumptions were true, they could not explain such a large weight gain. He concluded that lamb's wool stimulated the babies' skin more than cotton, and this stimulation probably reduced stress. Lowered stress, in turn, may have caused the babies to gain weight. Richards cited an intriguing parallel to this phenomenon in cultures that traditionally swathe infants.

At the monkey laboratory of the University of Wisconsin, scientists carried their research of touch several steps further. Psychologist Stephen

Suomi and his colleagues divided young monkeys into two groups. One group was separated from their mothers by a glass partition. Although the mothers and infants could smell, hear and see each other, they could not touch. In this group, some monkeys underwent short-term deprivation of touch. Others were separated from their mothers for longer periods.

The study's second group of monkey infants was similarly separated, but with a dividing screen between infants and mothers that could be penetrated. The degree of touch which they were allowed was enough to prevent serious long-term behavioral problems. For the monkeys in the first group who were deprived totally of touch, physical separation from their mothers had serious consequences. According to Suomi, those separated by the impenetrable glass partition for short periods spent " . . . too much time in intense physical contact with a partner. These animals will cling to one another as adolescents when such behavior is more typical of that of an infant. And spending all of this time clinging to one another, they have no time to spend in normal activities such as grooming, play or sexual sorts of interactions." For the monkeys deprived of maternal touch for longer periods, disturbed behavior was extreme. They tended to avoid other monkeys. Interactions that did occur, Suomi said, were often "uncoordinated and . . . exceedingly aggressive."

Current research has revealed that such problems are more deeply rooted than previously thought. Deprivation of touch, under certain conditions, can cause brain damage. Scientists at the University of Illinois separated monkeys into three groups. The first was allowed to interact naturally. Monkeys in the second group were individually isolated by a glass partition for twenty hours a day. For the remaining four hours, the glass was removed. Once the monkeys settled down, they interacted normally until separated again. In the third group, however, monkeys lived in total isolation. They could neither see, hear, smell nor touch one another. Later autopsy of their brain tissue, analyzed by computer, revealed structural damage to nerve cells of the cerebellum. The Illinois team was surprised to find

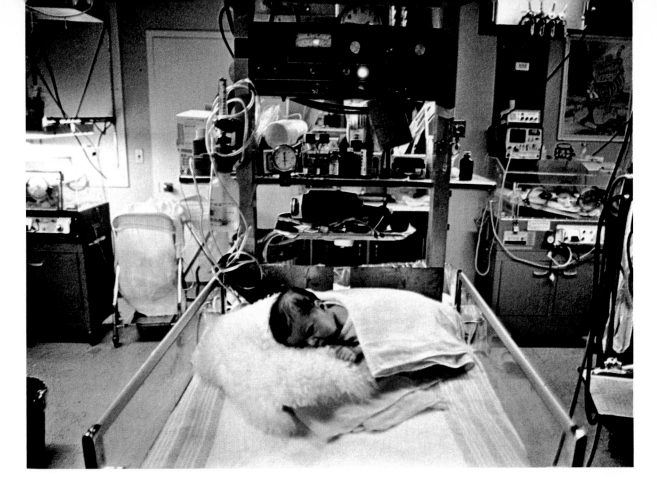

similar damage in the partially isolated monkeys. As the researchers expected, the first group suffered no damage whatever.

Scientists are just beginning to learn how touch deprivation affects people. Alexander Lowen, a psychiatrist, believes that schizophrenia can be caused by lack of intimacy between a mother and her child. "The lack of erotic body contact," Lowen maintains, "is experienced by the child as abandonment. If the child's demands for this contact are not met with a warm response, it will grow up with the feeling that no one cares." Several therapists have reported that massaging, embracing, tickling and caressing can sometimes break through the isolation characteristic of schizophrenic patients.

Lesser emotional problems may also be related to touch deprivation. At the Menninger Clinic in Topeka, Kansas, researchers observing emotionally disturbed young people have speculated they were denied touching as infants. Marc Hollender, a psychiatrist at the University of Pennsylvania, found that twenty-one of a group of thirty-nine patients had used sex in order to entice men to hold them. Hollender quoted a former prostitute who admitted, "In a way, I used sex to be held." Although Hollender did not investigate the early

histories of these women with regard to touching, another expert has suggested that touch was somehow denied them.

Recent experiments have revealed that touch influences human interactions in subtle ways. Richard Heflin, a social psychologist at Purdue University, instructed library clerks to touch some readers when returning their identity cards. Heflin carefully specified that the touch be both casual and fleeting. Later, readers were interviewed about their feelings toward the library. Those who had been touched reported more positive feelings. Heflin was amazed by his results, which he believes demonstrate that even the most insignificant touch can change a person's mood and perceptions. In another Purdue experiment, one of Heflin's students left a dime in a telephone booth. The student would approach the next caller, saying, "I think I might have left a dime in there. Did you find it?" Sixty-three percent of the callers returned the dime. When the researcher lightly touched the person, however, the return rate rose to 96 percent.

In another country, these experiments might have yielded far different results. Different cultures harbor different attitudes toward touching. Anthropologist Ashley Montagu noted that

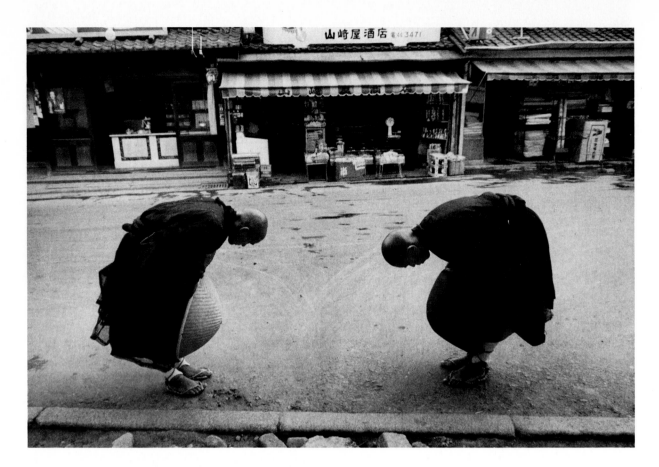

among Englishmen, "The public demonstration of affection was vulgar, touching was vulgar, and only men who were quite outside the pale — such as Latins, Russians, and the like — would ever dream of putting their arms around each other, not to mention indulging in such effeminacies as kissing each other on the cheek." "Crushed against his brother in the Tube," writer Germaine Greer once remarked of the London subway, "the average Englishman pretends desperately that he is alone." A different standard prevails in France, where passengers on the French Metro press against each other without embarrassment. Social scientists have confirmed these observations. One researcher watched pairs of people conversing in coffee shops in several different countries. In Puerto Rico, over a one-hour sitting, the people touched 180 times. In Paris, they touched 110 times. In London, there was no touching at all.

Americans are only slightly warmer than the cool English on the scale of touching. Within the culture, however, attitudes toward touching vary according to ethnic background. One researcher even found that touching can diminish as immigrant families become Americanized. Studying Roman Catholic families before and after church services, he found that Italian-Americans in an Italian section of Boston touched about every twenty-seven seconds. But in the middle-class suburb of Newton, the churchgoers touched about every forty seconds. Moreover, according to the researcher, the Boston Italians' touches "seemed more sincere and giving" compared to the more assimilated Newtonians.

Like touch, the use of space varies according to culture. Ashley Montagu observed, "While waiting for a bus, Americans will space themselves like sparrows on a telephone wire, in contrast to Mediterranean people who will push and crowd together." One researcher watching crowds at the Houston Zoo noticed that Mexican-Americans generally stood closer together than Anglo-Americans. Anthropologist Edward Hall found that Germans required wide personal space. Standing on a threshold or talking through an open door, which Americans find unthreatening, is an outrageous intrusion to a German. "In every instance," Hall declared, "where the American would consider himself *outside* he has already entered the German's territory." In 1965, psychologists Michael Argyle and Janet Dean proposed their "equilibrium theory" of interpersonal space. The theory proposes that people are attracted as

With elegant formality, Buddhist monks in Japan greet each other. Different cultures harbor vastly different attitudes toward touching. The Japanese, among others, prefer to keep their distance.

well as repelled by others, and use space accordingly. Once a proper distance is established, it is maintained. If one person leans away, the other leans forward, or compensates by smiling or making stronger eye contact. Other investigators studying how people space themselves in lines discovered that perfume and brightly colored clothing put more distance around the person wearing them.

A Question of Power

Space and touch establish rank and convey a sense of power. Psychologist Nancy Henley has studied and written about nonverbal communication. She tells one story about an incident at the University of Maryland, where she was teaching at the time. After a faculty meeting, the vice chancellor approached her, grabbed her upper arms and said he had something to discuss with her. When he had finished, she grabbed him back and told him about her research. She mentioned that touching established hierarchies and conveyed power. At that moment, the chancellor of the university came over, put his hand on the vice chancellor's arm, and said that they needed to leave for the next meeting. The chancellor was the only person on campus with a higher rank. "I think the point was aptly made," said Henley. Edward Hall suggests that a wide buffer zone is automatically established around important public figures. He cites Theodore White's *Making of the President, 1960.* When John Kennedy's nomination became a certainty, "others in the room surged forward on impulse to join him. Then they halted. A distance of perhaps 30 feet separated them from him, but it was impassable."

The intimate bond between touch and power is perhaps most dramatically forged in India, where 100 million people called untouchables lie at the bottom of the social order. Untouchables include fishermen, people who kill or dispose of dead cattle, sweepers and washermen. Traditionally, the touch of these people was thought to pollute those of higher castes. In southern India, even the sight of an untouchable was once thought polluting. Mahatma Gandhi tried to abolish this deeply entrenched system, calling untouchables *harijans* (children of the Hindu god Vishnu). Although

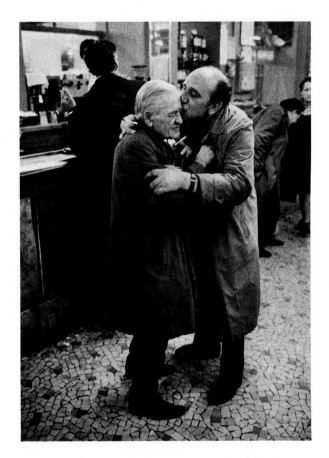

A friendly kiss and warm embrace mark greetings in France, even between men. Studies have shown that the French are more eager to touch in casual encounters than the English, who are cooler in public.

117

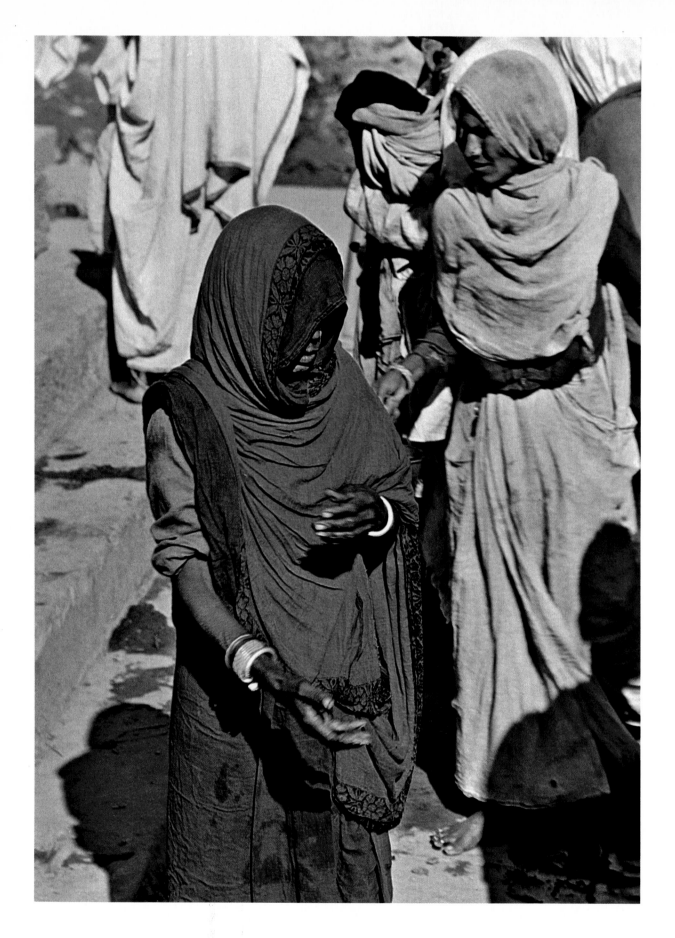

A forlorn beggar, one of India's
untouchables, gestures to passersby
near the Ganges. Under the Indian
caste system, the touch of such a
person is thought to pollute those in
higher castes.

banned by India's 1949 constitution, the custom is rooted in 3,000 years of Hindu history and stubbornly persists. One untouchable explained, "We are not allowed to carry our towels on our shoulders. We can't take water from a common well. We can't sit on a bench where a caste Hindu is sitting." Sometimes, attempts by low-caste Hindus to keep untouchables in their place erupt in violence. In late 1981, there was a massacre of untouchables in a village near the Taj Mahal. An Indian reporter wrote, "They killed the *harijans* like rabbits."

The Skin's Sensors

Their unenviable status notwithstanding, even the most wretched untouchables are blessed with the gift of touch. Amoebas, brushing against a particle, sense whether it is a foreign body. Touch is one of the least understood of man's senses. Minute corpuscles and receptors help us feel pleasure and pain, heat and cold, pressure and movement. Scientists are still divided over the precise workings of these organs in the skin. One thing, however, is certain. Without them, we are lost.

The largest receptors are Pacinian corpuscles. Attached to thick, fast-conducting nerve fibers, Pacinian corpuscles are onion-shaped sensors that lie deep inside the dermis. Nevertheless, they are exquisitely sensitive. Pressure on the skin of two ten-thousandths of an inch will arouse these corpuscles in one-tenth of a second. In cats, Pacinian corpuscles are concentrated in the paws, leg joints and connective tissue of the abdomen. This arrangement may be responsible for a cat's crouching posture. With the Pacinian corpuscles close to the ground, cats can quickly detect the movement of prey. Similar sensors on the snout of moles feed them information about soil. Closely related corpuscles on the tongues of woodpeckers help them find insects in tree bark. In man, Pacinian corpuscles lie not only in the dermis but around joints and tendons and in tissue that lines organs and blood vessels. Scientists believe the fast-reacting receptors provide instant information about how and where we move.

Lying between the dermis and epidermis are Meissner's corpuscles, egg-shaped capsules har-

boring a mass of intertwined fibers that branch out from a nerve terminal. Meissner's corpuscles are concentrated in the fingertips and palms, lips and tongue, nipples, penis and clitoris. This abundance is thought by scientists to lend special sensitivity to these regions. Meissner's corpuscles inform the body exactly where the skin is touched. Like other skin sensors, each controls an area called a receptive field. One experiment revealed that a Meissner corpuscle on a fingertip responded to a pressure of 20 milligrams, about the weight of a fly. If pressure was applied only eight-thousandths of an inch away from the center of the corpuscle's receptive field, however, the force needed to excite the sensor was ten times greater. Although not as fast to respond as Pacinian corpuscles, Meissner's corpuscles fire less than a second after triggering. Oddly enough, receptive fields seem to change over time. Sometimes they vanish altogether, while new ones are created. Scientists are at a loss to explain this baffling process.

Merkel's disks, flat, oval-shaped organs lying in the epidermis, are concentrated in fingertips and other areas where Meissner's corpuscles are found. Merkel's disks are usually arranged in bundles called Iggo dome receptors, which cause the skin to bulge slightly. The receptive fields for Iggo domes are so sensitive that they react to pressures of less than one-thousandth of an ounce. Unlike Meissner's corpuscles, Merkel's disks transmit a weak but continuous signal after their initial firing. Scientists therefore believe that these sensors are specialized for gathering information about continuous touch rather than movement across the skin.

Somewhat mysterious, Ruffini endings and Krause end bulbs are receptors that lie deep under the epidermis. Both are encapsulated by sheaths of connective tissue and contain lacy networks of nerve fibers. Researchers think they participate in man's ability to detect heat and cold as well as pressure. This would explain the paradox that cold objects feel slightly heavier than warm ones. Ruffini endings are also found in the joints, where they signal information about how far a joint has rotated. Krause end bulbs are concentrated in the lips, tongue, penis and clitoris. Ruffini endings lie deeper in the skin and are less widely distributed.

Grouped around the roots of hairs are nests of receptors for detecting movements. The slightest pressure on a hair sounds the alarm that the hair has brushed an object. Animal whiskers serve the same purpose. Recent experiments with rabbits, cats and monkeys have shown that displacement of a hair by as little as four hundred-thousandths of an inch can trigger these receptors.

Lacing the dermis are free nerve endings, which branch out endlessly to form an intricate web covering the whole skin. Free nerve endings are even found in the cornea, where they inform the eye of touch and pressure.

Scientists disagree on the role and function of the touch receptors. At the end of the nineteenth century, German physiologist Maximilian von Frey first articulated the now classical view that each receptor had a special duty. Under this classification, Pacinian corpuscles detect pressure; Meissner's corpuscles and Merkel's disks, touch; Ruffini endings, heat; Krause end bulbs, cold; and free nerve endings, pain. The research by Ainsley Iggo, discoverer of the structures that bear his name, tends to support the traditional view. In the 1950s and '60s, Iggo and his colleagues at the University of Edinburgh separated individual nerve fibers from bundles and traced them to the skin's surface. They then applied various stimuli to the skin to see how the fibers would react. Some fibers responded only to pressure, others only to temperature. Iggo also found that some fibers, particularly slow-firing ones, responded to more than a single sensation. Other researchers have noted that certain skin areas, including the ear, contain free nerve endings but few corpuscles. Nevertheless, the skin of the ear can detect all the sensations of touch, temperature and pain with accuracy.

These discrepancies have led some scientists to suggest the sensors of the skin are somewhat, but not completely, specialized. Supporters of this view note that receptive fields for different sensors often overlap, and that stimuli from the skin are carried to the central nervous system by fibers of varying thickness, affecting the speed at which signals are carried. These scientists believe that the distribution of impulses among small and large nerve fibers form a pattern which the brain recognizes as a particular sensation.

The most distressing sensation is pain, which Albert Schweitzer once called "a more terrible lord of Mankind than even death itself." Pain is Nature's warning system of injury — a unique and indispensable tool for survival. Although rare, congenital defects can leave babies numb to everyday pain. Such individuals live in great peril. Without the alarm signals of pain, they can suffer extensive tissue damage before noticing something amiss.

The Perception of Pain

Pain is a mixed blessing. Often, the sensation is wholly out of proportion to the injury. A mere pinprick can cause an intense, stabbing pain, but a lethal brain tumor may linger for months without producing the slightest discomfort. Nor does pain necessarily warn us of serious injuries. The victims of migraine headaches endure prolonged, deeply unpleasant pain without any head injury.

Despite important studies, scientists still do not know what really happens when we feel pain. Based on current understanding, pain seems to proceed something like this: Suppose you burn your finger on a hot kettle. Immediately, chemicals that inflame tissues called histamines and hormonelike chemicals called prostaglandins alert free nerve endings to the burn. Histamines and serotonin, a neurotransmitter released by blood cells, divert additional blood to the injury, producing external redness and swelling. This process is abetted by the adrenal glands. Alerted by nerves to the emergency, the glands release epinephrine, causing the heart to pump blood faster. Blood serves two functions at the site of the injury. First, it sweeps away the debris of damaged tissue. At the same time, it marshals supplies of fuel and oxygen to initiate repairs. Because blood is diverted to the burn, there is now less in the stomach and intestines. Digestion can slow down or virtually cease, depending on the severity of the crisis. Gastric juices stop flowing, and the smooth muscles of the intestine that push food along relax. Food stays in the stomach until the emergency passes.

Egg-shaped Pacinian corpuscles lie
beneath the skin and immediately
alert nerves to the slightest pressure.
Similar receptors on the tongues of
woodpeckers help them find insects
in tree bark.

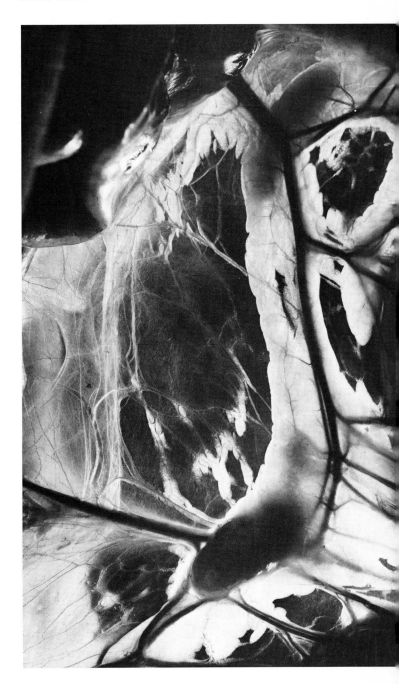

Pain travels to the spinal cord through two types of nerve fibers, one that transmits pricking pains and another that transmits burning and aching pains. Pricking pain signals travel at speeds between six and thirty meters per second. Burning and aching pains move more slowly, about one-half to two meters per second. This slow-lane, fast-lane approach explains why pricking pains are followed by a slow, burning pain. Each type of nerve fiber follows separate pathways through the spinal cord and the brainstem to the thalamus, the brain region that scientists believe serves as a terminal for decoding pain signals. At this stage, the picture becomes cloudy. Knowledge about pain is overwhelmed by questions begging answers. To their general astonishment, however, scientists are continuously discovering that the mind has remarkable control over pain.

Circumstances, it appears, play an important role. During World War II, Henry Beecher of the Harvard Medical School saw severely wounded soldiers in combat hospitals at Anzio, Italy. He was surprised to learn that only about one in three asked for morphine. When he returned to the United States after the war to practice as an anesthesiologist, Beecher asked patients whose surgical incisions resembled the soldiers' wounds whether they wanted morphine after their operations. Four of five patients claimed they were in severe pain and begged for a morphine injection. Beecher concluded, "There is no simple direct relationship between the wound per se and the pain experienced."

Other researchers explored the implications of Beecher's work and made more puzzling discoveries. Scientists in England found that when the word "pain" appeared in a set of instructions, anxious subjects were more likely to report an electric shock as painful. Researchers also found that severe pain can often be alleviated by giving patients a placebo, such as a saline solution, in place of morphine. In one experiment, roughly 35 percent of the patients given a placebo said they felt better.

Recent research suggests that people relieved of pain by placebos are actually manufacturing their own painkillers, a class of chemicals called

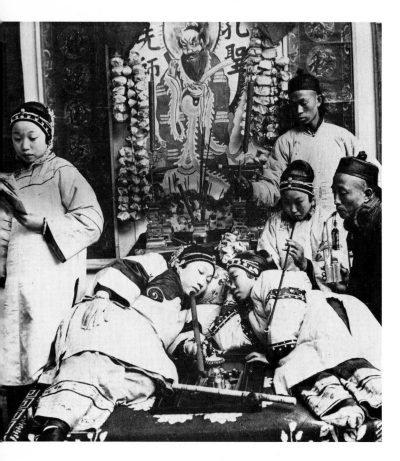

Intoxicated with opium, Chinese smokers lounge languidly in a den. Opium exerts its euphoric power by mimicking the action of endorphins, a group of body chemicals that are natural painkillers. Opium and its derivatives — heroin, morphine and codeine — occupy the same sites in the brain as endorphins.

endorphins — literally, "the morphine within." Manufactured by both the pituitary gland and the brain, endorphins are neurotransmitters that relieve pain naturally. They may also help control body temperature and affect consciousness. Morphine and other opiates, like heroin, are effective painkillers precisely because they mimic endorphins, by occupying the same receptor sites in the brain's nerve cells. Considering the power of their poppy-derived imitators, endorphins are potent indeed.

Describing his first experience with opium in *Confessions of an English Opium Eater,* nineteenth-century writer Thomas De Quincey exulted, "Here was a panacea . . . for all human woes: here was the secret of happiness, about which philosophers had disputed for so many ages, at once discovered: happiness might now be bought for a penny, and carried in the waistcoat pocket: portable ecstasies might be had corked up in a pint bottle: and peace of mind could be sent down in gallons by the mail coach." Scientists believe that opiates cause the body to temporarily shut down production of the painkilling endorphins. The resulting lack of natural opiates sets up addiction and withdrawal. De Quincey also described withdrawal, writing, "Think of me as of one, even when four months had passed, still agitated, writhing, throbbing, palpitating, shattered."

The painkilling effects of both morphine and endorphins can be quickly reversed by another drug called naloxone. Naloxone occupies the same receptor sites in brain cells as opiates and endorphins but, for unknown reasons, does not trigger the same painkilling effects. Naloxone can push opiates off the receptor sites. This property has made naloxone a standard fixture in hospital emergency rooms, where many overdosed heroin addicts have been rescued from comas by timely injections. Solomon Snyder, the director of the Department of Neuroscience at Johns Hopkins University, has reported seeing, "overdosed heroin addicts, deep in a coma, recover within fifteen seconds of receiving a naloxone injection."

Using naloxone as a tool for detecting endorphins, researchers at the University of California at San Francisco tested fifty patients recovering from wisdom tooth operations. Some were given morphine to kill pain, some a placebo and the others, naloxone. As expected, about a third of the patients who received placebos reported less pain. When this group was then given naloxone, they said the original degree of pain had returned. Naloxone's only known effect is to block endorphins (and their imitators, heroin and morphine). Researchers concluded that the placebo had caused the patients to psychologically boost their own production of endorphins.

If learning and expectation affect the perception of pain, so apparently does culture. Bush doctors in East Africa still perform an operation called trephination on patients with incurable headaches. The doctor first prays for success and then slices away the scalp with a crude blade. He removes a chunk of skull and replaces the scalp over the hole. Through the procedure, even with his brain exposed, the patient shows no sign of distress or pain. It is a phenomenon that mystifies scientists.

The East Africans are not alone in their seeming indifference to pain. American artist George Catlin described a religious ceremony, *O-kee-pa,* which he witnessed among the Mandan Indians of the Upper Missouri River in 1832. According to Catlin, the annual event ensured that the Mandans would find buffalo to hunt, and failure to strictly observe the tradition " . . . would bring upon them a repetition of the calamity which their traditions say once befell them, destroying the whole human race, excepting one man, who landed from his canoe on a high mountain in the West." *O-kee-pa* included torture to prepare young warriors for manhood and to help the chiefs decide who would be worthy of leading war parties. Tribal elders cut incisions through the skin on the shoulders, hands, arms, legs and chests. Wooden splints attached to ropes were inserted into the incisions. From all but the shoulder and chest splints, buffalo skulls, shields or medicine bags were hung. The men were then lifted off the ground with the ropes attached to their shoulder or chest splints. Despite the gruesome ritual, the men only expressed pain when, once suspended, they were twisted in the air. When the initial incisions were cut, according to Catlin, the warriors "beckoned me to look them

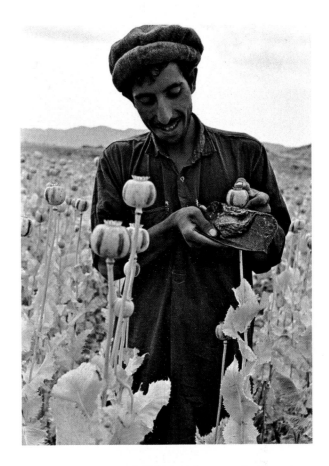

A Pakistani farmer cuts an unripe capsule of the poppy, the source of opium, to collect its milky juice. Sometimes called crude, the air-dried juice contains anhydrous morphine, a highly addictive narcotic agent.

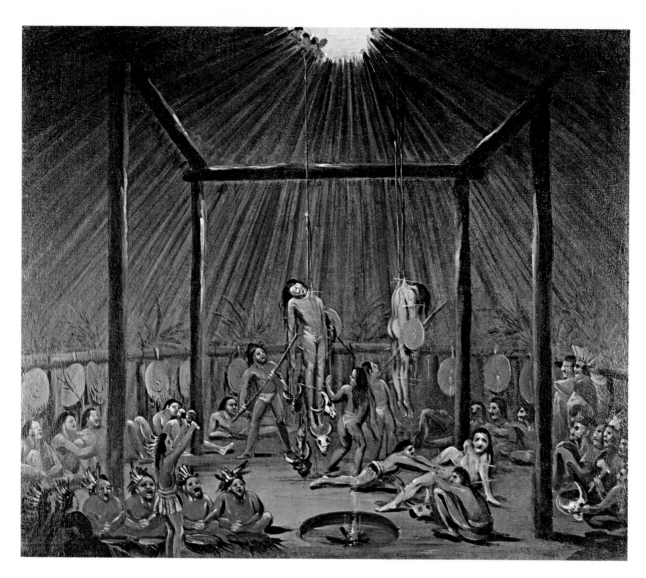

Stoic Mandan warriors undergo a
tribal torture ceremony in this
painting by nineteenth-century
American artist George Catlin. The
ritual's purpose was to find men best
suited to lead war parties, based on
how well they withstood the agony
of the ordeal. The men were suspended by ropes attached to splints
passed through their shoulders and
chest. When their flesh was pierced
for insertion of the splints, they
expressed little pain.

in the face, and sat, without the apparent change of a muscle, smiling at me whilst the knife was passing through their flesh, the ripping sound of which, and the trickling of blood over their clay-covered bodies and limbs, filled my eyes with irresistible tears."

Scientists do not know why an African can calmly endure brain surgery without anesthesia or why a Mandan could smile while his flesh was cut open. One hypothesis was recently advanced by two researchers who conducted comparative tests on porters in Nepal and camel drivers in Algeria, people accustomed to hard labor and pain. The researchers concluded that although they felt pain, "culturally imposed stoicism" prevented them from complaining.

Whatever the merits of this theory, simple stoicism cannot explain the puzzling phenomenon of fire walking. The Roman scholar Pliny noted that a Roman family, at an annual sacrifice to Apollo, would "walk over a charred pile of logs without being scorched." Similar feats are still performed in India, Spain, Japan and Thailand. In the small mountain village of Kosti in northern Greece, fire walkers celebrate the miracle of St. Constantine, who is believed to have saved sacred icons from a flaming church in 1250. The Greek villagers first meditate in the room where the icons are kept and perform a ritual dance. During the actual fire-walking ceremony, they walk on white-hot beds of coals, sometimes kneeling for several minutes.

Nor can science explain couvade, the practice of a husband feeling labor pains while his wife gives birth. In some cultures, a woman about to have a child will work in the fields until she goes into labor. Her husband then takes ill and groans while she bears the child. The woman almost immediately returns to attend the crops while the husband recovers from his trauma by resting in bed with the newborn baby at his side. Although anthropologists have devised elaborate explanations for couvade, many researchers believe that sympathy pains are real. In Western countries, similar pains are not uncommon. One man recalled that during his wife's pregnancy, he felt sick in the morning and had chills. Another father remembered, "I woke up every morning

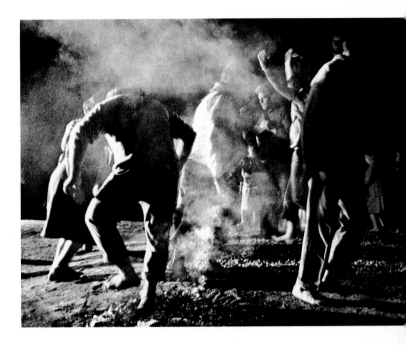

Greek villagers from the mountain town of Kosti dance across red-hot coals. The fire-walking ceremony commemorates St. Constantine, who rescued icons from a burning church in 1250. Scientists are unable to explain why the men feel no pain.

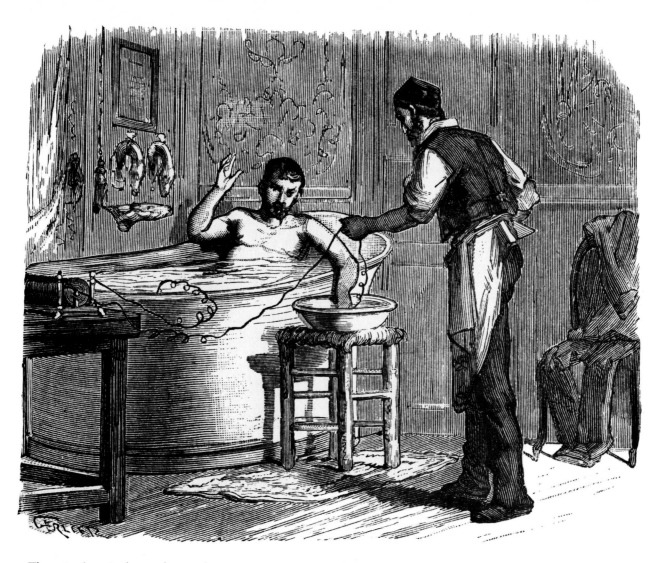

Therapies for pain have a long and occasionally bizarre history. This treatment, called the electric bath, was probably never popular but seems to have enjoyed a momentary appeal at the turn of the century.

from the fifth month of my wife's pregnancy with nausea —like a mild hangover.''

People sometimes feel pain where there cannot be pain — a phenomenon called phantom limb. French physician Ambroise Paré described it in 1552, declaring, ''Verily it is a thing wondrous strange and prodigious, and which will scarce be credited, unless by such as have seen with their eyes, and heard with their ears, the patients who have many months after cutting away of the leg, grievously complained that they yet felt exceeding great pain of that leg so cut off.'' Most amputees report feeling phantom limb soon after amputation. In many cases, the feeling persists for years without discomfort. Others, however, develop lingering pain. One researcher talked with a woman who felt her phantom hand was tightly clenched, with the fingers digging into her palm. The pain vanished only when she was convinced that she could stretch her fingers open.

If science someday sheds light on these medical mysteries, still another hurdle must be overcome — helping people in chronic pain. For most people, pain is fleeting, unpleasant and quickly forgotten. But for many, as Thomas Hardy wrote in *The Mayor of Casterbridge,* happiness is "but the occasional episode in a general drama of pain." Chronic pain is the third largest health problem in America. Migraine headaches, slipped disks and arthritis afflict millions. The months or years of suffering commonly begin with surgery, an accident or an illness. For some victims, every moment is spent in almost unbearable pain. Many cannot sleep, and most are unable to work. The average pain patient has endured three operations and has as much as $100,000 in medical bills. The habitual use of painkillers carries a grave risk — addiction.

Searching for breakthroughs in the battle against chronic pain, researchers have developed powerful painkilling drugs which, unlike morphine, are not addictive. Among them is Zomax, a pain reliever approved by the Food and Drug Administration in 1980. Georgetown University professor of pharmacology William Beaver called Zomax "one of the most impressive compounds for pain developed so far." The drug interferes with the body's production of prostaglandins, chemicals crucial to the transmission of pain to the brain. In trials with cancer patients, Zomax was found as effective as morphine.

Another promising type of therapy is the transcutaneous nerve stimulator (TNS). A 1960s outgrowth of cardiac pacemaker technology, transcutaneous nerve stimulators are portable, battery-powered machines that send electronic signals through the skin, giving some relief to perhaps 70 percent of chronic pain patients. Some scientists believe the electronic signals block pain messages from reaching the brain, while others believe that they boost the body's production of endorphins. Because the device uses large amounts of power, researchers have been hampered in their efforts to develop models that, like pacemakers, can be implanted beneath the skin — without the need for constant battery changes. Scientists at the Johns Hopkins Applied Physics Laboratory are now working on building

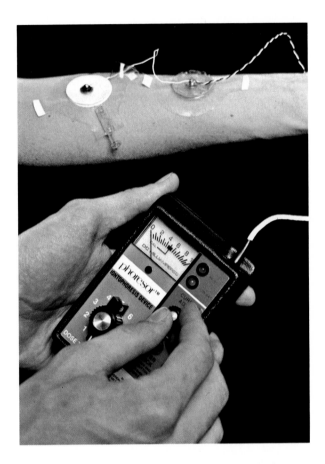

Science intercepts pain with the transcutaneous nerve stimulator (TNS). An outgrowth of 1960s cardiac pacemaker technology, TNS sends electric currents into the skin, bringing pain relief to 70 percent of chronic pain patients.

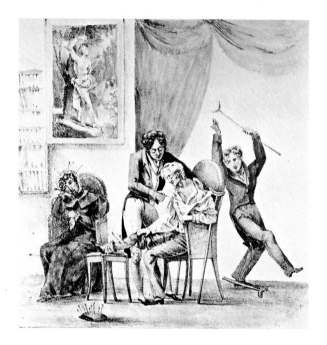

While another patient is treated with needles, a previously ailing man celebrates his restored health through "the marvelous effect of acupuncture" in this satiric French lithograph from the nineteenth century. Practiced for at least 7,000 years in China, acupuncture was introduced to the West by Jesuit missionaries in the seventeenth century. In Europe and America, it remained the work of quacks until the mid-twentieth century.

miniaturized stimulators that can be recharged outside the body.

Many pain patients say they experience relief from biofeedback and hypnosis. Biofeedback machines, monitoring muscle tension with electrodes, allow the patient to learn how to relax. "The patient can hear, see and feel muscle tension," declared one specialist. After practicing on the machine, patients learn how to recreate the feelings that offered relief. Similarly, hypnosis enables patients to recreate the moods of a trancelike state that helps them control pain.

While some chronic pain victims are finding relief in these new techniques, others are turning to acupuncture, an approach thousands of years old. Scientists believe that acupuncture has been practiced for at least 7,000 years. Early needles from the Neolithic Age in China were made of flint and bone. The earliest documented evidence comes from the Chinese medical text, *The Yellow Emperor's Classic of Internal Medicine,* which was based on ancient oral traditions and written in the third or fourth century B.C. By that time, metallic needles were widely used. Gold and silver acupuncture needles were among the finds from a tomb in Hebei Province dating to 113 B.C.

In traditional Chinese medicine, acupuncture needles are inserted into the skin at strategic points and twisted. The ancients believed that the body was a sort of energy field with lines of force called currents that moved along certain routes. Acupuncture points were stations along these routes. Today, acupuncture is sometimes practiced in China to deaden pain during surgery. Often, electric currents are channeled through the needles, eliminating the need for relay teams of nurses to twist the needles. Initially skeptical, Western scientists have become convinced in the past decade that acupuncture works. Its precise mechanism remains unknown, however. At the National Institute of Mental Health, researchers have conducted experiments that suggest the technique somehow boosts the production of endorphins, the body's natural opiates. Chinese doctors who practiced the ancient art for centuries might not have been interested in such an explanation. They believed in what they saw — the relief of pain.

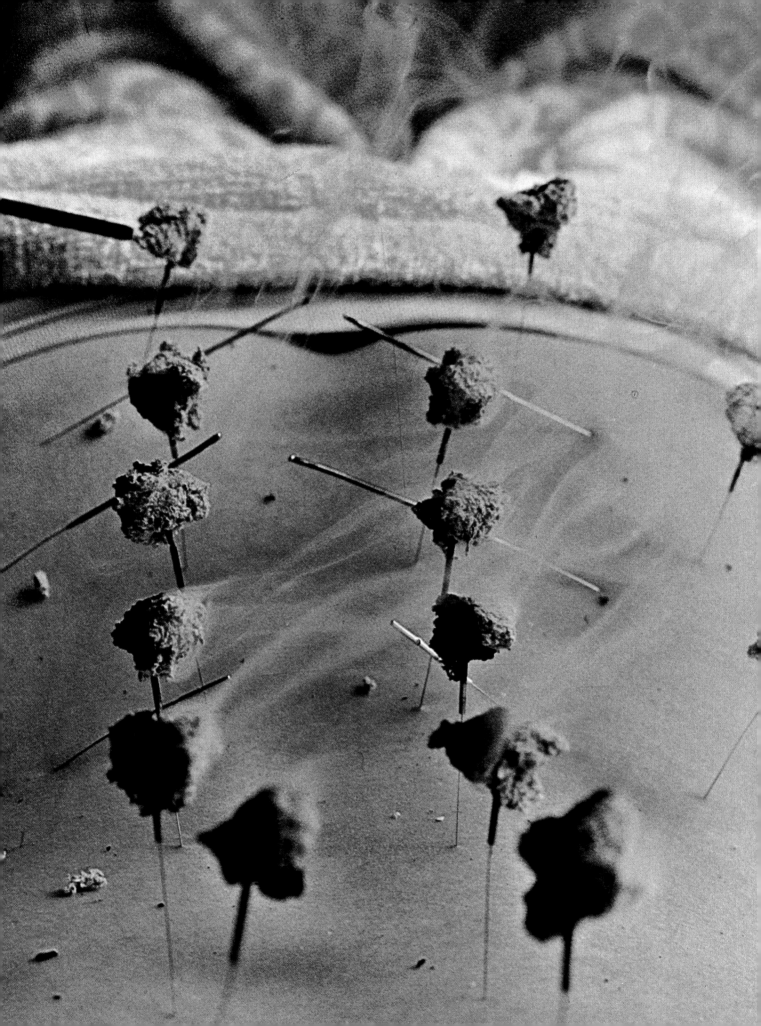

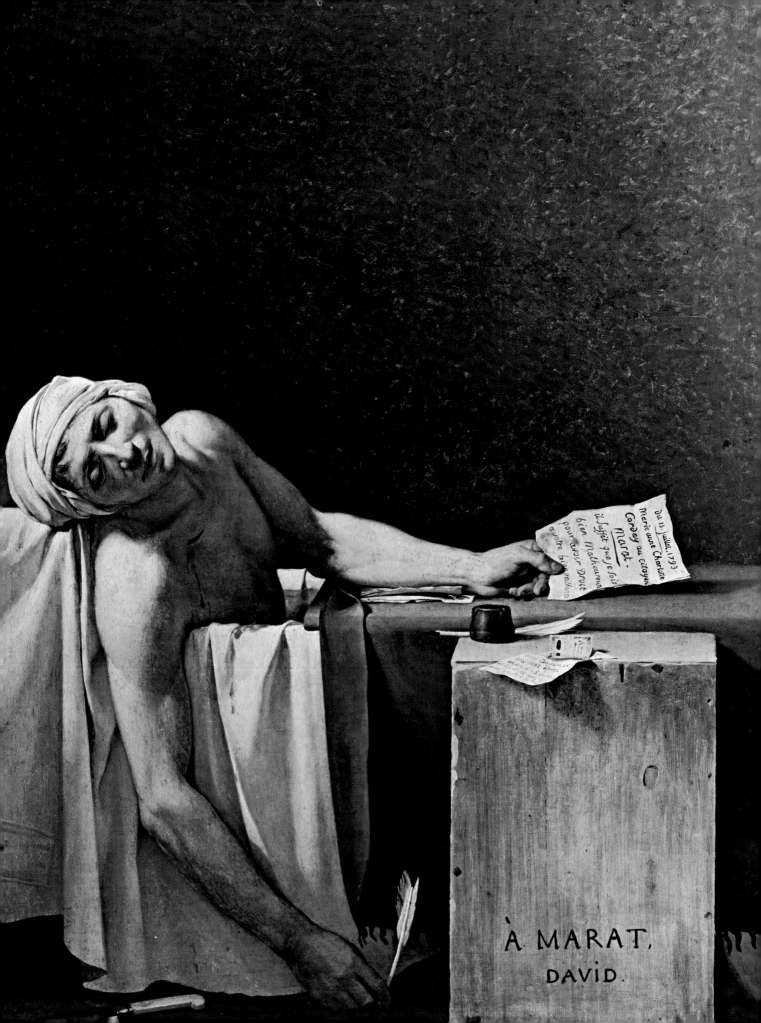

À MARAT,

DAVID.

Chapter 6

A Thousand Natural Shocks

eauty's but skin deep," observed a poet of Elizabethan times — a depth, actually, of only a few millimeters. This thin, elastic covering gloves the body from scalp to sole, giving color and character to the human form. Of all the body's tissues, none is more exposed to disease and injury than the skin. Viruses and bacteria may infect it. Allergic reactions to sun, drugs and food can inflame it. Internal changes may damage it. The skin is assaulted by a thousand traumas, by bites and stings, burns and blisters, rashes and pocks, by moles and warts and all.

The siege begins in infancy and continues all through life. Moles, called pigmented nevus cells, often occur soon after birth and tend to increase until early adulthood. Then they usually begin to fade, and in old age may vanish altogether as they are worn away by the body's immune system. Tan macules freckle sun-loving youngsters, especially those with red hair and fair complexions. Senile lentigines, dark macules commonly known as "liver spots," typically appear on the sun-exposed foreheads and the hands of older persons. Nevus cells take many forms, and some may disfigure the body or become malignant. While freckles and beauty spots are best admired instead of treated, melanomic nevi generally should be surgically removed.

Such childhood blemishes doubtless gave man his first evidence of the skin's vulnerability, but leprosy was an infectious wasting of the skin that filled him with dread, for it carried the stigma of uncleanness, unrepented sin. Now known as Hansen's disease, it has scourged civilizations since the dawn of history. The Bible, in the Book of Leviticus, defines the ill: "When a man shall have in the skin of his flesh a rising, a scab, or bright spot, and it be in the skin of his flesh like the plague of leprosy . . . and when the hair in the plague is turned white . . . the priest shall look on him, and pronounce him unclean." The

Jacques Louis David's masterpiece The Dead Marat *portrays the martyrdom of revolutionist Jean Paul Marat. Afflicted with the skin disease dermatitis herpetiformis, said to have been contracted while he hid in the sewers of Paris, Marat sought relief by soaking in a hot tub. On July 13, 1793, an assassin gained admittance on a ruse and stabbed him in his bath.*

131

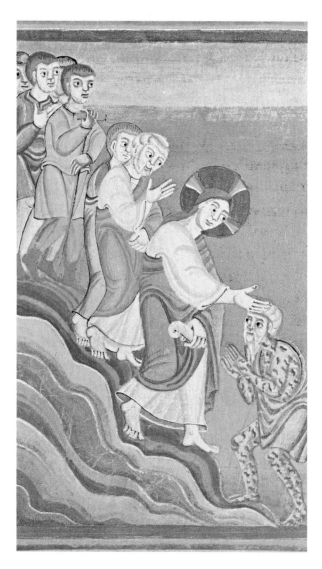

"Stand up and go on your way," Jesus commands a leper in the New Testament's Luke. "Your faith has cured you." Such scripture inspired this eleventh-century illumination from Echternach Gospels Lectionary.

individual was declared a *metzorah,* a "leper," and isolated. Priests looked for other changes as well, such as erosion or an increase in size. Following the progress of the sore, they would set conditions of ritual impurity. If the lesion healed, the patient went through a ritual cleansing that included immersion and sacrificial offerings.

Tzaraat, the biblical term for leprosy, has no modern counterpart. Historians speculate that over the centuries *tzaraat* may have represented stages of several diseases or was perhaps changed through competition with other infectious maladies. One theory holds that the spread of pulmonary tuberculosis "could have interrupted the infectious chain" of leprosy by providing some degree of immunity.

One study of more than 18,000 skeletons suggests that leprosy did not exist until the sixth century, despite the fact that houses for lepers had been established in Europe two centuries earlier. Roman rulers, perhaps influenced by Christian ideals, began taking seriously biblical injunctions to separate persons with disfiguring skin ailments — perhaps syphilis, psoriasis, vitiligo and other disorders as well as true leprosy.

Leprosy made its way into southern Europe from the Near East, first by coastal traffic on the Mediterranean and, later, by Crusaders returning home. In 379, St. Gregory of Nazianzus condemned lepers as "men already dead except to sin; often dumb, with festering bodies whose insensible limbs rotted off them . . . objects of repugnance and terror." Rothar, king of Lombardy in the seventh century, decreed that a leper should be expelled from his home and be "considered as dead." Five hundred years later, the leper was symbolically buried in medieval masses that sequestered him from the unblemished faithful. Stripped of all dignity, he knelt beneath a black cloth as a priest ceremoniously spilled spadefuls of cemetery earth on his head and commanded: "Be dead to the world, be reborn to God." In England, the first king of the house of Anjou, Henry II, punished lepers for their sins by burning them at the stake. Philip V of France soon adopted Henry's solution.

Fearing contagion, the church invoked the injunction in Leviticus that lepers "shall dwell

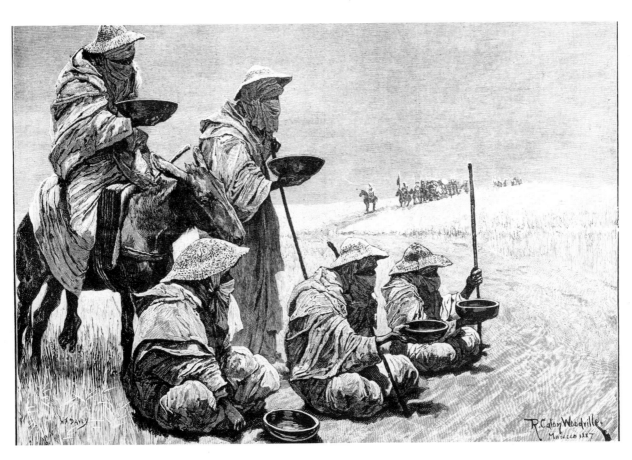

alone, without the camp," and banished them to leprosariums beyond town walls. Monasteries of St. Lazarus became known as lazarhouses or lazarettos. By the end of the thirteenth century, 19,000 of them sheltered "Christ's poor," as lepers were called. Within the asylums life was grim. One book of rules described leprosy as the most loathsome of diseases and stipulated that "those who are smitten with it ought at all times, and in all places, as well as in their conduct as in their dress, to bear themselves as more to be despised and as more humble than all other men."

Franciscan monk Bartholomeus Anglicus — Bartholomew the Englishman — observed that the flesh of a leper "is notably corrupt" with "many small botches and whelks. . . . The nails are boystous and bunchy, the fingers shrink and crook." And "in the body be diverse specks, now red, now black, now wan, now pale. The tokens of leprosy be most seen in the utter parts . . . in wasting and minishing of the brawns of the body." The monk unhesitatingly recommended a cure: "To heal or to hide leprosy, best is a red adder with a white womb, if the venom be away, and the tail and the head smitten off, and the body sod with leeks, if it be oft taken and eaten."

Proscriptions of the times against the leper were many. He was forbidden to wash in a stream, enter a tavern, walk in a narrow lane (lest he meet another person) or eat with anyone but lepers. If a person spoke to him, he was obliged to put himself downwind before replying. He was not allowed to leave his house without donning the leper's costume. Although styles varied from place to place, he traditionally wore gloves and a long robe — often black with a red *L* embroidered on it. He carried a rattle or a bell to warn others of his approach, and a stick to point with. Sometimes a mask covered his face, and a pair of horns yoked his shoulders.

133

Father Damien

A Saint Among Outcasts

"Damien, crowned with glories and horrors, toiled and rotted in that pigsty of his under the cliffs of Kalawao." So wrote Robert Louis Stevenson of the Flemish priest who spent the final sixteen years of his life working among lepers on the Hawaiian island of Molokai.

Born Joseph De Veuster in 1840, he adopted the name Damien as a nineteen-year-old novice, convinced that "God wishes me to leave the world to embrace the religious life."

Spring of 1863 found him in Honolulu, one of a group of missionaries. Jubilantly he penned a letter: "Here I am, dear Parents, a missionary in a land corrupt, heretical, idolatrous. . . . Do not forget, I beg you, the poor priest who day and night will be tramping about the volcanoes of the Sandwich Islands in search of stray sheep."

Little did Damien dream then that the flock he sought would be a colony of lepers confined to Kalawao, a rock-strewn promontory of Molokai hemmed in by high cliffs and the sea. Many of its wretched occupants, loath to leave homes and families, had been forced to the leprosarium. Police flushed them out of hiding and herded them aboard the ship that was to ferry them to the island.

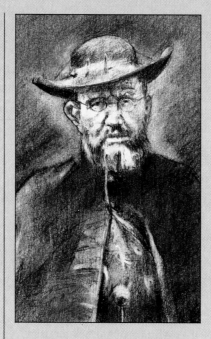

On such a ship, Damien arrived. What he saw appalled him: a few grass huts, a rude hospital without medicine or beds, lepers "running about in tatters . . . the sick wallowed in frightful dirt."

Damien stepped ashore "bent on devoting my life to the lepers." He took shelter under a pandanus tree until he scrounged enough lumber to build a small cabin. As the catechism instructs, he set about feeding the hungry, clothing the naked, caring for the sick, and burying the dead. He became carpenter, policeman, banker, nurse, beggar, confessor for a parish population that often numbered close to a thousand.

Wielding hammer and saw, he built homes for the living and coffins — some 1,600 of them — for the dead. He often dug the graves, as well.

He strove to banish idleness, inspiring the sick to plant crops and organize games. One musician fashioned a piece of wood to replace missing fingers, enabling her to continue playing the harmonium, an organlike instrument.

Even before he contracted leprosy, Damien identified with his parishioners, saying, "We lepers . . ." By the early 1880s it was apparent that he was seriously infected. "Soon I shall be completely disfigured," he wrote. "But I stay calm, resigned, and quite happy in the midst of my people." A few years later the words were more doleful: "I have been steadily yielding the last flickers of vitality, and I have drawn much nearer to the cemetery." "My face and my hands are already decomposing." By the time he died, a few days before Easter in 1889, he had become "the most repulsive leper in the lazaretto."

A legend, he lived as a saint among outcasts. Said one witness: "I have seen him dress the most loathsome sores as if he were arranging flowers."

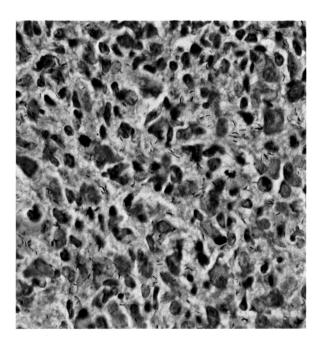

Rodlike microbes of the bacillus Mycobacterium leprae *abound in magnified tissue from a mangabey monkey. In this primate and the armadillo, researchers are seeking a vaccine for leprosy.*

Segregation of lepers and victims of other diseases considered contagious became a widespread medical practice. In Ragusa, the medieval port in Yugoslavia now called Dubrovnik, an isolated area away from the harbor was reserved for new arrivals suspected of carrying infectious disease. Individuals were held for a *trentina* — thirty days. Later extended to forty days, the period of isolation became known as *quarantina.* Quarantining lepers, however, was an ineffective measure.

The disease is communicable only after prolonged exposure — usually within the immediate family. Even so, 90 percent or more of adults in close contact with lepers prove to be resistant to the infection. What causes leprosy? Some 2,100 years ago, in *Nei Ching,* the Manual of Physics, Chinese physicians postulated "winds and chills lodge in the blood vessels and cannot be got rid of." In the *Midrash Rabbah,* a collection of interpretations of the Old Testament begun in the second century, Hebrew scholars cited all manner of wickedness, including the seven abominations to God in Proverbs:

Proud eyes, a lying tongue,
Hands that shed the blood of the innocent,
A mind full of evil schemes,
Feet running toward wrong;
A false witness breathing out lies,
And one who stirs up quarrels between brothers.

Some medieval thinkers suspected that the consumption of goat's milk and rotten fish induced leprosy. Friar Bartholomew theorized that "it comes of corrupt meat as of measled hogs," and he warned against prolonged use of pepper and garlic. The "evil is contagious," he moralized, believing the disease was communicated through sexual intercourse, for "it cometh of flesshely lykynge by a womman soone after that a leprous man hath laye by her."

According to the church, the mark of leprosy was neither an impediment to marriage nor was it a cause for divorce. Pope Gregory IX decreed in the thirteenth century that "spouses must not be separated from marriage because of leprosy." Nevertheless, when the church declared a leprous wife symbolically dead, the husband could decide he was free to remarry.

The risk of becoming infected with leprosy as a result of conjugal contact or prolonged exposure is not as great as medievalists feared, for most persons are not susceptible to the disease. Those prone to leprosy likely contract it through the mucous membranes of nose and mouth or by means of skin abrasions.

In 1879, several centuries after leprosy had run its virulent course throughout Europe, Scottish surgeon Sir Patrick Manson discovered rodlike microbes in "leper juice" extracted from patients' lesions. But Manson was unable to grow the bacilli in a culture — a hen's egg. Six years earlier, Norwegian doctor G. Armauer Hansen had been convinced that the bacillus could be transmitted from one host to another. He resorted to experimentation on an unwilling subject. Pricking the eye of a woman, he infected it with the substance from a leper's nodules. Hansen stood trial for his unethical conduct and was let off with a reprimand. Ironically, his name became synonymous with leprosy, but without the stigma of the unclean outcast.

Although 90 percent of the world's population may be immune to leprosy — and even patients are noninfectious if the disease is controlled by drugs — an estimated 13 million cases exist, more

135

than 8 million of them in Asia. Africa accounts for 3.5 million. Over the last twenty years, the number of cases in the United States has increased fivefold, to about 4,200, due largely to the influx of refugees from Third World countries. The National Hansen's Disease Center in Carville, Louisiana, where lepers were once forcibly detained, admits patients today on a voluntary basis. They are free to leave at any time. About 125 patients live at the leper settlement on Molokai, Hawaii, the last admitted in 1969.

At Carville in 1941, a medical milestone was reached when the sulfone drug dapsone was successfully used to treat leprosy. Although slow-acting, often having to be administered over a lifetime in order to remain effective, dapsone was inexpensive, costing a patient only about $2 a year. India annually uses fifty tons of the drug. But there and elsewhere, dapsone alone has failed to arrest drug-resistant strains. Other drugs, notably those used to fight tuberculosis, have proved effective against leprosy, but they cost up to 300 times more than dapsone. World Health Organization investigators are attempting to solve the problem with combinations of drugs.

Researchers continue their century-long quest for a vaccine. In 1960, Charles C. Shepard, head of the leprosy lab at the U. S. Centers for Disease Control in Atlanta, Georgia, found that the footpads of mice provided an environment for the proliferation of the bacillus. A more useful model for experiments lay almost at the door of Carville laboratories — the nine-banded armadillo. The armor-plated mammal proved to be a reliable incubator of leprosy bacteria, possibly because of its low body temperature, which is several degrees lower than most other mammals' and matches the temperature of human limbs. At the Dermatological Institute in Caracas, Venezuela, researcher Jacinto Convit inoculated several hundred leprosy patients with a serum derived from bacteria cultivated in armadillos. Combined with a tuberculosis vaccine, the treatment resulted in apparent cures within eighteen months.

Some researchers believe that vaccinating millions of people would be excessively expensive because the odds of contracting leprosy after exposure are so low and the incubation period in humans is three to six years. Thus, a decade or more would have to elapse before a significant reduction in the disease could be determined. Treatment with drugs, it is argued, could wipe out leprosy more efficiently.

"Tell me O God — how long?" a leper's poem laments. The deliverance from leprosy is a dream of uncounted centuries that promises to become reality. The discovery of leprosy in monkeys during the 1970s could further man's understanding of the disease. But other diseases of the skin, many once lumped with leprosy, persist.

Too Many Cells
Psoriasis sufferers have long been plagued by patches of thickened, scaly skin. Stages of the disease range from a few isolated lesions to erythroderma — a widespread redness of the skin. The disfigurement is caused by runaway production of new cells in the epidermis, the skin's outer layer. Imperfectly formed because of accelerated growth, the immature cells flake from the skin like crusty dandruff. Psoriasis lesions are readily recognized, but doctors occasionally perform biopsies or patch tests to rule out other inflammations. Rarely covering the entire body, psoriasis appears most often on the elbows, scalp, knees and lower back. The itching lesions cause mental anguish as well as physical discomfort.

Flexural psoriasis, a common form of the disease, appears in folds and creases of the skin rather than on larger areas. Guttate psoriasis — from the Latin *gutta,* meaning "drop," shows on the skin as scattered spots. Generalized psoriasis, rarely seen, occurs when painful inflammation covers the body. During attacks, sufferers undergo changes in body temperature and lose water through the skin. Psoriasis can pit or separate fingernails and change their color.

No one pattern emerges from the many studies of the disease's origin, but it appears that this ailment generally runs in families. One study found a higher incidence of psoriasis among identical twins than among fraternal twins, leading scientists to believe that certain individuals are genetically predisposed to the disease. They suspect that several genetic factors probably dictate if and how psoriasis is inherited.

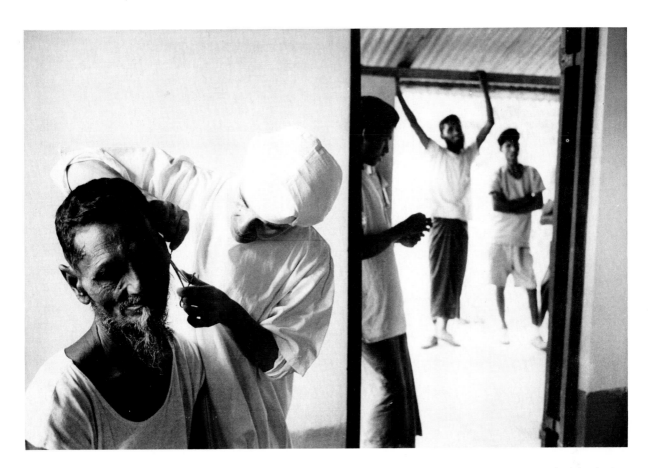

Corticosteroids, anti-inflammatory agents that suppress the immune system, and methotrexate, a drug that reduces the cellular production of a certain acid, are administered to psoriatic arthritic patients. Common psoriasis is treated with various corticosteroid ointments. These compounds, chemically related to the hormone cortisone, improve scaly patches in half the patients who use them. However, the administration of steroids in any form — topical, oral or intramuscular — should be monitored by a physician for side effects that range from infection to acne.

Ultraviolet treatment for psoriasis was first developed in the early twentieth century by an American doctor. Still popular, the Goeckerman treatment, named after its inventor, consists of applying a coal-tar preparation to the skin, washing it off, then exposing the skin to ultraviolet rays. A more recent treatment combines the use of light-sensitive plant substances known as

Sister Solange Bernard snips dead skin from a patient in a leper colony at Jalchatra, Bangladesh. The ages-old disease plagues more than eight million Asians. They are treated with the sulfone drug dapsone, developed in 1941 at the National Hansen's Disease Center in Carville, Louisiana.

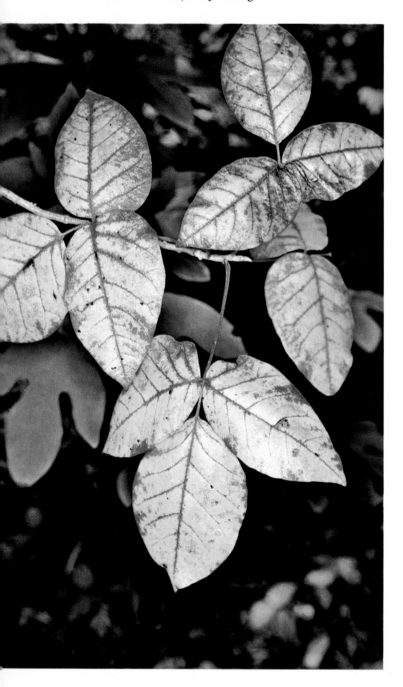

Its trifoliate leaves bronzed by autumn, poison ivy is a bane to most who touch it. Washing with detergent soon after contact may prevent skin from blistering. Commercial lotions relieve temporary itching.

psoralens (P) with exposure to ultraviolet light (UVL) in the longer wavelengths of the A range — thus the acronym PUVA. According to Ernesto Gonzalez, a dermatologist and expert on psoriasis at Massachusetts General Hospital, "PUVA is not a cure, but a maintenance treatment. Seventy-five percent of the cases we handle require treatment every week or every other week." PUVA has been spectacularly effective in treating psoriasis. On occasion, it appears to cause skin tumors. Such tumors are easily excised, however, and Gonzalez maintains, "The benefits of PUVA far outweigh any risks."

The body has many sophisticated responses to chemicals both within and outside it. These responses can present themselves as allergy and as autoimmune disease. Allergy causes inflammation in response to a foreign substance, or allergen. Skin reaction in autoimmune disease occurs because the body's natural defense system turns against a substance of the body. Autoimmune disease is thus an expression of allergy to self.

Scleroderma, or systemic sclerosis, is a generalized disease of the connective tissues. It can affect any organ in the body, most noticeably the skin, which loses elasticity and becomes hard like armor plate. The hardening results from the body's collagen replacing the subcutaneous fat. A disease that remains a mystery to researchers and physicians, scleroderma has no known cause or cure. The patient — most often a female between twenty-five and fifty-five — lives with periodic episodes of exacerbation and remission.

Another mysterious disease of possible autoimmune origin is vitiligo, a pigmentation disorder involving the skin cells that produce color. When these melanocytes are destroyed, white patches appear on the skin. Vitiligo responds to a varied arsenal of drugs. PUVA treatment appears to give some patients periods of remission.

Triggered by both allergy and irritant, contact dermatitis is a rash that accounts for 10 percent or more of all patients admitted to hospitals. A rash may appear immediately after contact with an allergen, or it may not show up until days later. Urticaria, commonly called hives, may occur after a sensitized person takes a hot bath, eats chocolate or strawberries or inhales spores from a moldy basement. The list of allergens in both hives and contact dermatitis is long.

Physicians sometimes have difficulty distinguishing between allergic contact dermatitis and that caused by irritants. The following situation illustrates the two reactions. A family wears clothes washed in a detergent. Each family member experiences an irritating rash. When the mother exposes her skin to a new perfume, she breaks out in a second rash. Her daughter applies the same perfume but does not react to it. Throughout the day the mother contends with symptoms ranging from runny nose and watery eyes to excessive sneezing. She has reacted both to an allergic and an irritant contact dermatitis.

Substances causing the rash are contactants. An unusual rash appeared on several patients living in the New York-Connecticut area. The rash, resembling poison ivy, had never been seen before by doctors. The contactant causing it turned out to be the larvae of the gypsy moth. The wind-borne larvae dropped on unsuspecting humans, causing hives, pain in the respiratory tract and insomnia brought on by the itching. Some patients eventually required oral steroids.

Leaves of Three

An estimated three-fourths of the American population is allergic to poison ivy and its companions — poison oak and poison sumac. Belonging to the genus *Rhus*, all can cause severe dermatitis. "Leaves of three, leave them be," warns the children's rhyme — and for good reason. Susceptible persons can become infected after strolling in the woods or weeding the garden. Even handling gardening tools that removed the noxious plants can transmit the allergen. Pet a dog that chased a rabbit through poison ivy, and you may find blisters on the palm of your hand within forty-eight hours. The blisters usually disappear within two weeks if the oil, a toxic oleoresin, is not spread by scratching. Washing contaminated skin with soap within ten minutes of exposure may prevent the blisters from forming.

Folk remedies for poison ivy abound. A salve to relieve itching is made from the orange sap of jewelweed. Also called touch-me-not, it is often found growing in damp, shady areas near *Rhus*

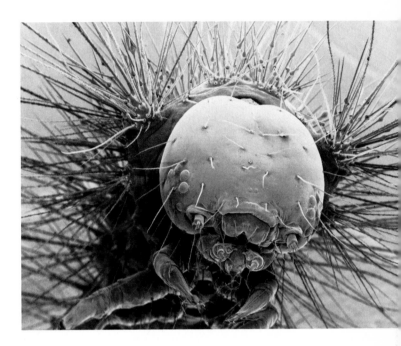

As fierce as it looks, the gypsy moth caterpillar attacks humans as well as trees. Contact with its sharp fiberglasslike bristles, which are laden with histamine, causes a skin rash similar to the dermatitis poison ivy inflicts. Some victims who react severely to its touch may experience shortness of breath, as well.

139

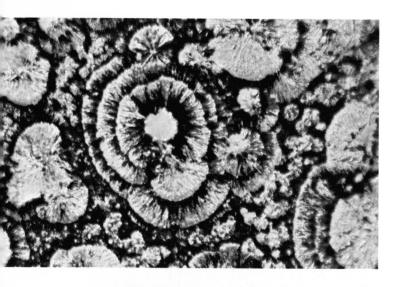

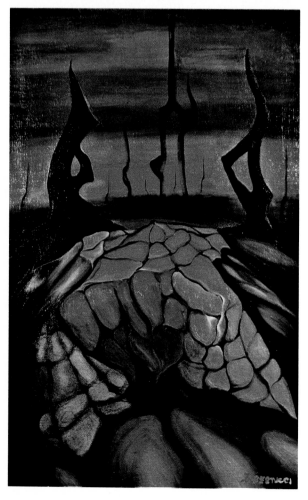

plants. American Indians used goldenseal to promote healing, bathing inflamed skin with a solution of the yellow-rooted herb. Juice from the leaves of aloe vera, a succulent frequently grown as a house plant, is said to lessen swelling.

Hot water stops the itching for sixteen-hour intervals. Adding baking soda or cornstarch to water often reduces the discomfort. Many medicine cabinets contain the time-honored standby, calamine lotion. Corticosteroid preparations are also effective when applied locally. In severe cases, steroids are injected or taken orally.

A more serious form of contact dermatitis afflicts persons exposed to the chemicals Agent Orange and formaldehyde. Agent Orange is a defoliant used against North Vietnamese and Viet Cong troops in Southeast Asia that has caused toxic skin reactions, weight loss and cancer. Formaldehyde, introduced into the environment by shampoos and cosmetics, foam insulation, auto emissions, cigarette smoke and industrial smog, can irritate eyes, skin, nose and throat.

People who work on farms may be subject to "noninfective" dermatitis. Causes, according to the *British Journal of Dermatology,* include extremes of climate, barley dust, mites that feed on grain causing "straw or barley itch," pesticides and herbicides and antibiotics administered to animals. As the use of chemical agents increases on today's high-technology farms, workers face more dermatologic hazards.

A major cause of disability to miners is so-called occupational dermatitis, caused by dust. Prolonged exposure under cramped working conditions causes "a wear and tear type of eczematous dermatitis," a study in England determined. "One might regard it as a cumulative insult," noted the report. A panel of British doctors concluded that persons susceptible to eczema and other skin disorders should not work in mines.

Eczema, related to irritant and allergic contact dermatitis, has been described as atopic in nature, meaning "out of place" or "strange." Caused by the body's reaction to common foreign substances, such as intolerance to milk or allergies brought on by pollen, the disease's "boiling out" — from the Greek word *ekzein* — occurs when blood vessels ferry allergens to the skin.

There, a battle takes place between allergens — also called antigens — and antibodies, protective substances secreted by tissues. Locked in combat, they cause inflammation characterized by intense itching. If the reddened patch is scratched, infection is likely to develop, with the skin oozing and bleeding and becoming encrusted.

Many infants develop seborrheic eczema, a form of dandruff called cradle cap that affects the scalp and skin around the ears. Itchy "milk crusts" cover baby cheeks. Some physicians believe that milk-protein hypersensitivity often lies at the root of infantile eczema. However, after the age of two the chief agents that trigger sensitivity are not foods but materials like wool, feathers, dog or cat hair and human dander.

Infection superimposed upon the eczema comes from invading staphylococcal and streptococcal bacteria. Untreated infections can lead to swollen lymph glands, yellow crusting and kidney disease. The combination of staphylococcal and streptococcal infection can cause skin disorders such as impetigo. This pustular eruption appears on hands, feet, scalp and extremities. Highly contagious, patients with impetigo must avoid physical contact with other people.

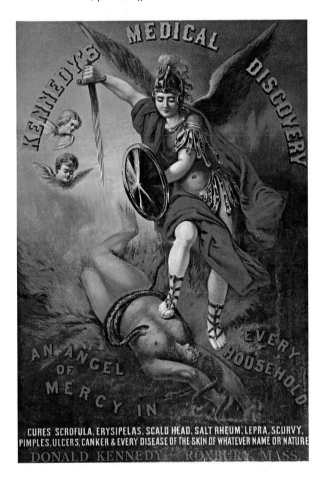

A time-honored prescription for impetigo, *Eau Dalibour,* dates from about 1700 when Jacques Dalibour, surgeon general to Louis XIV, compounded a solution containing copper and zinc. It was beneficial not only for skin eruptions but for "all Manners of Wounds, Cuts, Slashes by Sword or Sabre, and Injuries by all Cutting and Bruising Devices." Infectious complications of eczema such as impetigo are now treated with a variety of antibiotics, especially erythromycin.

While some skins are intolerant of drug therapy, others cannot tolerate sunlight. By dilating blood vessels in the skin, sunburn causes inflammation. A photosensitive reaction to ultraviolet light may exacerbate viruses in the skin such as herpes simplex, trigger autoimmune diseases like lupus and precipitate sunstroke.

Medications may produce increased sensitivity to sunlight. Coal-tar derivatives, psoralens and antihistamines can cause allergic reactions to the sun. Oral sensitizers include antimicrobials such as tetracycline and sulfonamides. Doctors treat most photosensitive reactions with cortisone medications, which control the symptoms.

For another skin ailment, Mark Twain's Tom Sawyer proclaimed this cure: Dip your hand in a rotten stump filled with rain water and say:

Barley-corn, barley-corn, injun-meal shorts,
Spunk-water, spunk-water, swaller these warts.

Tom assured Huck Finn that "the wartiest boy in town . . . wouldn't have a wart on him if he'd knowed how to work spunk-water." He claimed to have rid himself of thousands of warts he got while playing with frogs.

Bacon fat is said to have cured Francis Bacon of warts when he visited Paris in the sixteenth century. The wife of the British ambassador rubbed on the fat, then nailed the bacon to a window frame. As it rotted, Bacon's blemishes disappeared. Other folk remedies include Irish potatoes, copper, snails, spittle, ink, a dead man's hand and deep thinking.

Scientists have long been fascinated by the power of the mind over such matter as warts. A professor of medicine used to assure his patients that warts painted with the dye gentian violet would disappear within a week — and they did.

Hypnosis works like a charm. One study shows the deeper the trance the better the chance that warts will disappear. They do so painlessly, without leaving scars and without the risk of the hypersensitive reaction local applications can produce. The main disadvantage of hypnosis, one researcher concluded, is the "considerable public and professional prejudice against [it]."

"Some intelligence or other knows how to get rid of warts," mused Lewis Thomas, chancellor of Memorial Sloan Cancer Center in New York, "and this is a disquieting thought. It is also a wonderful problem, in need of solving. Just think what we would know if we had anything like a clear understanding of what goes on when a wart is hypnotized away. We would know the identity of the cellular and chemical participants in tissue rejection, conceivably with some added information about the way viruses create foreignness in cells. . . . Best of all, we would be finding out about a kind of superintelligence that exists in each of us."

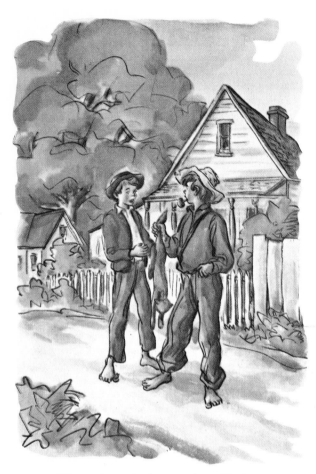

"Say—what is dead cats good for, Huck?"

Tom Sawyer asks Huckleberry Finn what dead cats are good for. "Cure warts with," he is told. But Tom knows something better — spunk-water found in a rotten stump. As Mark Twain's hero sensed, warts can apparently be charmed into disappearing, often by hypnosis. Most people, however, have them removed surgically rather than trusting the power of suggestion.

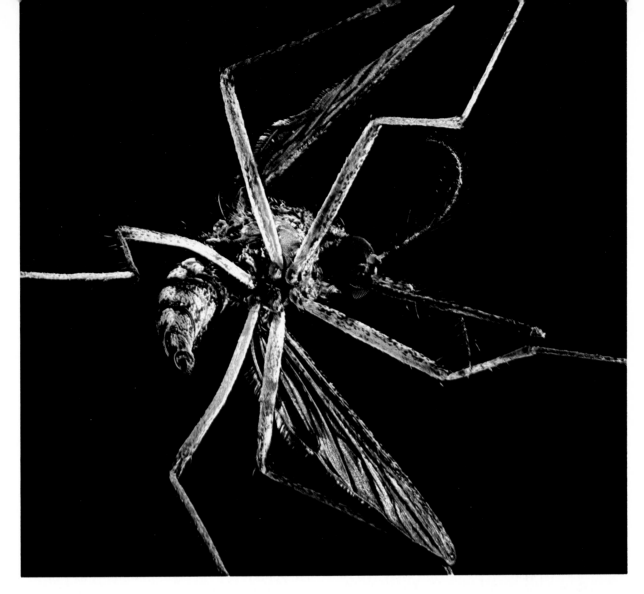

What we do know about the wart is that it is a manifestation of an infectious disease of the skin. It is caused by a virus that alters the DNA and causes epidermal cells to proliferate. These proliferations are classified by structure and location on the body.

Common warts occur singly or in clusters on the hands. Larger plantar warts usually infect the soles of the feet. Covered with a horny shell, they can be confused with corns and calluses. A dermatologist examines skin ridges to determine the difference. The ridges of a callus are continuous, while a wart's are uneven and broken.

Smooth, skin-colored flat warts stipple chest, neck, forearms and shins. Filiform warts appear as horny protrusions on the bearded areas of a man's face. Digitate warts form on the scalp and resemble little moles. *Condylomata acuminata* warts favor moist areas of the body, most often around the genitals. They are painful, can be numerous and should be distinguished from skin cancer and venereal diseases. Treatments include surgery and burning off warts with needle electrodes.

Time and loving care is the cure for the common blister, an annoying skin condition typically caused by ill-fitting shoes that rub against toe or heel. The accumulation of fluid under the top layers of skin is a reaction to excessive friction. Draining provides relief, but the covering skin should not be completely removed.

Painful swelling often results from insect bites and stings, sometimes with severe reactions. If the victim feels a general weakness or if his skin turns pallid or hives break out, prompt medical treatment should be sought. In most cases, first-aid measures suffice. These include applying ice packs, taking antihistamines and rubbing on meat tenderizer containing papaya enzyme. A slice of onion is said to lessen the pain of bee stings. The bites of mosquitoes and ticks can in-

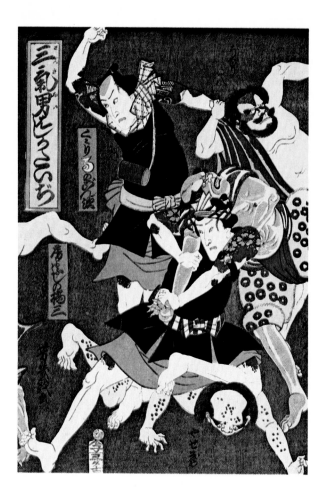

Measle demons pummel a victim to inflict the disease upon him in this Japanese woodblock print. The red spots appear on the skin after a patient develops fever, cough and a runny nose. A mild childhood disease, measles can be prevented with a vaccine of weakened measles virus or with gamma globulin injections soon after exposure.

fect the skin with bacteria that cause severe diseases. Newly discovered Lyme disease — named after the town in Connecticut — is transmitted by deer ticks. Beginning as a skin rash, it may develop into meningitis or arthritis.

As Lyme disease made its unwelcome debut, another malady that affects the skin was being stamped out. Measles, or rubeola, a virus infection once so common in towns and cities that almost every child broke out with the characteristic red rash, has all but vanished in the United States. Since 1941, when about a million cases were reported, systematic immunization has reduced the incidence of the disease to less than 14,000 by 1980.

As in many childhood diseases, fever, cough and runny nose mark the onset of measles. After a few days, red spots cover the patient. Although usually self-limiting and harmless, measles can sometimes become associated with secondary infections that lead to croup, bronchitis and pneumonia. Injections of gamma globulin within five days of exposure prevent the disease. A vaccine of weakened measles virus confers immunity.

Less contagious German measles, rubella, mainly afflicts schoolchildren of lower elementary grades. The rash, paler than that of rubeola, begins on the forehead and, like measles, spreads downward to cover the trunk and limbs. The lesions remain about three days. Pregnant women exposed to rubella may still transmit the virus to their fetus despite large doses of gamma-globulin serum. Prospective mothers are cautioned to avoid inoculation with live rubella vaccine, because it has the potential to cause birth deformities such as cataracts, deafness, heart defects and mental retardation. Vaccinations have been administered in the United States since 1969, producing a degree of immunity from German measles in nine out of ten cases.

Another disease common to children is chicken pox, or varicella. Highly contagious, it infects some 70 percent of those exposed. Adults may also contract it, but they experience a more severe rash and have a greater risk of developing pneumonia. During the course of the infection, tiny red-ringed lesions filled with clear fluid erupt, then dry to form scabs that fall off without scarring. As the disease evolves, various stages of the pox appear simultaneously on the body — mainly the trunk but also on the face and scalp. Tepid baths relieve the itching of chicken pox.

The same virus causes varicella and herpes zoster, or shingles. A disease of the nerves of the skin and the tissues surrounding them, herpes zoster typically attacks adults who had chicken pox as children. It is suspected that the virus lies dormant in spinal nerves until reactivated, probably through exposure to chicken pox or, occasionally, through zoster itself. Patients with malignancies, especially Hodgkin's disease, frequently develop shingles. Studies indicate that high doses of the antiviral protein interferon may benefit zoster patients, whose bodies have lost the ability to fight infection.

A Most Terrible Pox

On May 8, 1980, mankind triumphed over one skin disease. The World Health Assembly, which monitors inoculation programs, announced that "the world and all its peoples have won freedom from smallpox." Except for small reservoirs of the virus variola major in research laboratories, this most infectious disease in all history had been eradicated.

Thomas Macaulay, in his *History of England,* called smallpox "the most terrible of all the ministers of death." It had decimated London in the seventeenth century and taken even higher tolls on the Continent. With no respect for class or privilege, it felled Voltaire and Maria Theresa, empress of Austria — both of whom recovered — and France's King Louis XV, who did not.

Spanish conquistadors introduced smallpox to the Americas in 1520. It ravaged Indians and, later, colonists. In a letter to Patrick Henry during the War of Independence, George Washington declared smallpox "more destructive to an army in the natural way than the sword, and I shudder whenever I reflect upon the difficulties of keeping it out." The American siege of Quebec, some historians believe, was blunted not so much by the forces of Governor Guy Carleton as by the disease. "Our misfortunes in Canada are enough to melt the heart of stone," noted a congressman. "The smallpox is ten times more terrible than the

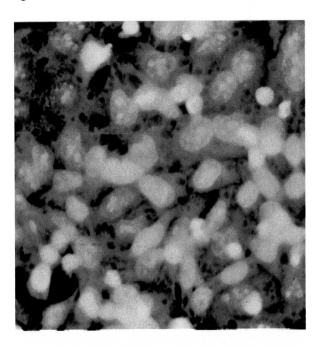

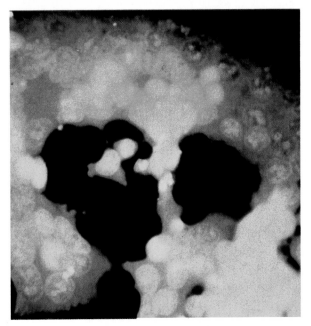

British, Canadians and Indians together. This was the cause of our precipitate retreat from Quebec." Washington apparently agreed, for the following January he directed his chief medical officer to inoculate the troops.

"Buying the pox" had long been practiced in the Old World. It was a method of variolation — after the Latin *varus,* meaning "pimple" — in which pus from an infected person was scratched into the skin of a healthy recipient. The inoculation usually produced a mild form of the disease, with a mortality rate of only about 10 percent of that normally associated with smallpox.

An eighteenth-century Boston physician combined variolation with pills, powders and bleeding, which was "conducted with a good deal of gayety." He ordered patients "to abstain entirely from animal Food, and all Kinds of Oil or greasy Substances, Salt, Spice, or Spiritous Liquors, great Fatigue and violent Exercise, together with all intense Thinking, and Application to perplexing Business." A twelve-year-old patient recorded in his diary, "Thus, through the mercy of God, I have been preserved through the Distemper of the Small Pox which formally was so fatal to many Thousands. . . . I should have a thankful Heart for so great a Favor. I confess I was undeserving of it. Many and heinous have been my Sins but I hope they will be washed away."

Variolation, lifesaver that it was, had a major drawback. When inoculated, a person became a carrier of virulent smallpox, which could be transmitted to others. There were exceptions. Fair-skinned English milkmaids who contracted cowpox — a benign, nonscarring disease transmitted from the teats and udders of cows — did not "take the smallpox" if they were variolated. The maidens appeared to be immune.

Edward Jenner, an English country doctor, believed that cowpox was a mild form of smallpox, and that inoculation with material from cowpox pustules could provide immunity without risk of contagion. In 1796, Jenner removed material from a pustule on the hand of dairymaid Sarah Nelmes and introduced it into the arm of James Phipps, "a healthy boy, about eight years old." From *vacca,* Latin for "cow," he dubbed the dairymaid's lesions vaccine disease — a learned way of saying cowpox. Inoculation of the material, which made the youngster immune from the effects of smallpox, became known as vaccination. Jenner rightly predicted that "the annihilation of smallpox must be the final result of this practice."

Before vaccination had halted its consuming course, smallpox spread from one contaminated person to another. Fever, malaise, headache, abdominal pain and blotchy redness heralded its presence. Pocks formed after the fever subsided. As the lesions spread, secondary infections set in, frequently causing death. Modern vaccination tools include a high-speed injector gun developed by the U. S. Army and a bifurcated needle that holds a drop of vaccine between the prongs. Before vaccine was refrigerated or preserved in dried form, an infected calf would be led door to door, providing fresh pus for each vaccination.

Unusual skin conditions are caused by many factors, some of them infectious, others genetic. Two diseases of genetic origin are ectodermal dysplasia and neurofibromatosis. Classified as phakomatoses — from the Greek *phakos,* meaning "lentil," "mole" or "freckle" — they combine neurological abnormalities with congenital defects of skin and other organs, areas often marked by nevi. Congenital ectodermal defect is characterized by loss of hair, malformation of teeth and malformation or absence of sweat glands. A genetic disorder, the disease may impair victims mentally as well as physically.

"Turtle Folk"

The "Whitaker Negroes," legendary subject of an essay by English poet and critic Robert Graves, were afflicted with this unusual skin problem. "The face was a glazed greenish-white, with four fangs that crossed over the lips," reads the description of a victim. His dark hair dripped water, and he wore large canvas gauntlets on his hands and sloshed about in leather brogans. His body smelled "as if fifty cess-pools had been opened."

The man was said to be a descendant of slaves bought by Mississippi plantation owner George Whitaker from pirate Jean Lafitte. Whitaker was mortified when he saw that the diseased Africans were useless as field hands. After drawing up a will, legend says, he and his wife jumped into the

146

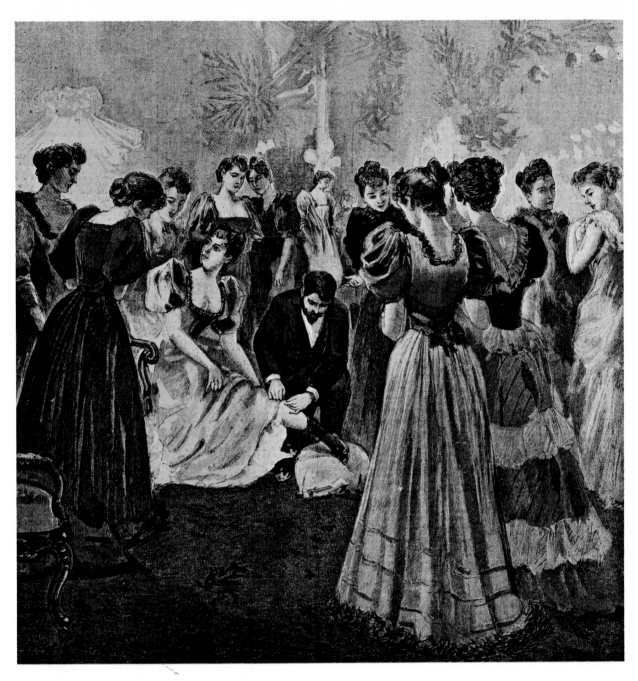

Mississippi River and disappeared. The slaves stayed on in the swamp, some marrying Indians. "The kids," noted Graves, "live in wallows under their huts, which are built on piles; apparently they don't come out much until they're fourteen years old or so — can't stand the sun.... The adults make a sort of living by raising hogs and chickens." The dripping hair turned out to be "mostly spanish-moss clapped wet on the head to keep it cool.... The brogans and gauntlets were filled with water. You see, they have no sweat glands . . . and their skin needs to be kept wet all the while, or they die."

There are other people without sweat glands called "turtle folk" by the local Mississippians. One mother keeps a tub of water handy in which to duck her young son. He, like other sufferers of this extremely rare disease, must be submerged periodically, like a turtle.

Perhaps the most grotesque of skin ailments is neurofibromatosis, or von Recklinghausen's disease, after the German pathologist who described it. Neurofibromatosis was little known until Ashley Montagu described it in *The Elephant Man*, a book which depicted the life of Joseph Merrick, an Englishman who was monstrously deformed

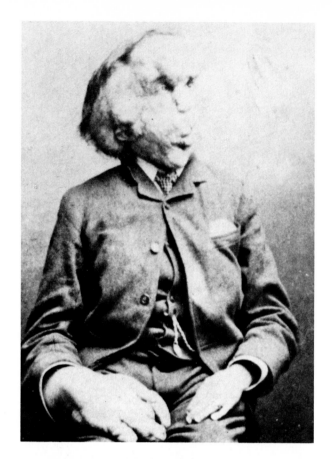

Gnarled features of Joseph Merrick, inspiration for Broadway's The Elephant Man, *were caused by neurofibromatosis. Werewolf tales sprang from porphyria victims with excessive facial hair, lower right.*

by the disease. "The most striking feature about him was his enormous and misshapen head," noted Frederick Treves, the physician who cared for Merrick. "From the brow there projected a huge bony mass like a loaf, while from the back of the head hung a bag of spongy, fungous-looking skin, the surface of which was comparable to brown cauliflower."

The disease affects one in every 3,000 live births. Patients may have no physical symptoms for years, with the exception of café-au-lait spots on the skin. The disease can range from cosmetic problems to life-threatening ones. Some patients have thousands of tumors. On rare occasions, the tumors become malignant. Merrick's face, said his doctor, resembled "a block of gnarled wood." His misshapen body forced him to rest his head on his knees in order to sleep. But in his desire to be "like other people," he apparently lay on his back, which crushed his spinal cord, and died.

Neurofibromatosis is a genetic disease passed from parent to child, affecting males and females equally. It may also be caused by a spontaneous genetic mutation. Lynne Courtemanche, co-founder of the National Neurofibromatosis Foundation and herself a victim of the disease, says parents are "appalled to learn their children have the disease because they have given it to them." She recommends that families receive psychological support. The only treatment for neurofibromatosis is removal of tumors by surgery, but the lesions sometimes reappear.

It is hoped that research being conducted by the National Cancer Institute will provide new answers for neurofibromatosis patients. Until that time comes, believes Courtemanche, they will have to draw strength from Merrick's example. He "bore up with tremendous dignity and grace," she says. "You have to develop an inner peace with yourself — otherwise you're just condemned to a living hell."

The same could be said for a rare congenital disease called porphyria, caused by an excess of naturally occurring substances called porphyrins, building blocks of the blood protein hemoglobin. Porphyria causes extreme sensitivity to sunlight. The build-up of porphyrins in teeth causes them to assume a reddish hue. Inexplicably, victims of

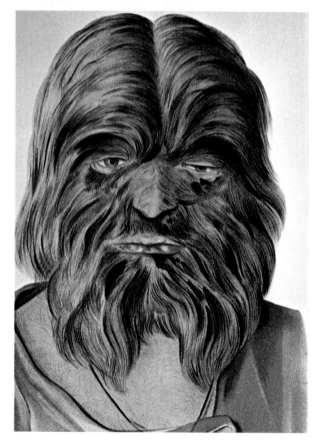

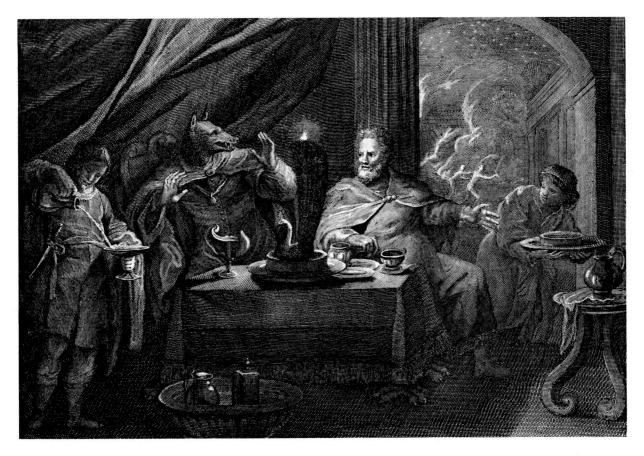

porphyria can sometimes suffer from hypertrichosis — excessive facial hair. Some scientists believe that these bizarre symptoms — red teeth, hairy faces and the need to avoid daylight —gave rise to legends of werewolves.

Myth and disease mingle in the Roman poet Ovid's account of a werewolflike figure: "In vain he attempted to speak; from that very instant His jaws were bespluttered with foam, and only he thirsted for blood, as he raged among flocks and panted for slaughter. His vesture was changed into hair, his limbs became crooked; A wolf, he retains yet large traces of his former expression. Hoary he is as afore, his countenance rabid, His eyes glitter rabidly, the picture of fury."

Universal folklore abounds in other ominous references to men changing into wolves. In the Middle Ages, suspected werewolves were sometimes flayed alive, as frenzied men searched for the wolf skin thought to lie beneath the human

one. James I of England deeply believed in the spirit world and noted in his treatise *Daemonologie* that the "warwoolfe" suffered from a "naturall superabundance of melancholie."

Although certainly not the cause of porphyria, melancholy would be an understandable result. Other symptoms include patchy inflammation of the skin, reddish urine in infants, pigmentation of the skin and ulcerating skin lesions, with eventual mutilating scars on the fingers, nose, eyelids and ears. These disfigurations, coupled with the appearance of facial hair, would easily arouse a fear of werewolves in a superstitious medieval peasantry. Treatment of porphyria is mainly preventive — avoiding sunlight. The application of sunscreens has proved of little value. Removal of the spleen sometimes lessens the side effects of anemia and photosensitivity.

Disfiguring as they are, inherited skin disorders generally are not life-threatening. However,

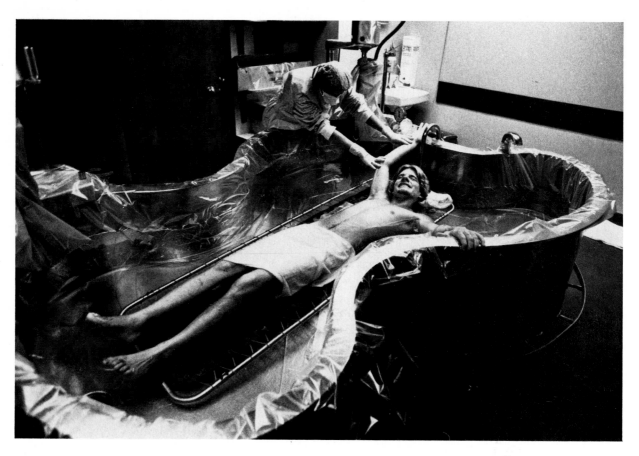

Recovering from second-degree burns over most of his body, a patient lies partially submerged in a tank while a therapist helps him exercise arms and shoulders. Filled with 100-degree water, the curved stainless-steel bathtub maintains a patient's body temperature as nurses remove charred tissue and cleanse wounds.

those caused by burns frequently do prove fatal. The third leading cause of accidental death — first, for persons under the age of forty — burns hospitalize at least 200,000 Americans every year. If the burn patient survives the risk of infection while undergoing massive antibiotic therapy, skin grafts, hot soaking and forced feedings, he may be faced with hours of physical therapy and psychological trauma.

The development of burn centers with highly specialized intensive care has decreased the mortality rate. Patients under the age of forty-five with burns on two-thirds of their body have a 50 percent chance of surviving. In dealing with the problems of infection and fluid loss, most crucial to the burn victim, the Albert Einstein College of Medicine in New York reports success with the chemical mercaptan N-acetyl cysteine, a drug that allows the process of grafting to be initiated quickly, after the removal of dead skin.

A new synthetic product, a polymer hydrogel, permits gas exchange, fluid regulation and the absorption of antibiotics as it shields burned skin. This also speeds up the grafting process and lessens the risk of infection. Burn centers and hospitals rely heavily on a silver sulfadiazine cream, Silvadene, which is used in dressings that are changed every day, an excruciatingly painful experience for the patient. One nurse encourages her patients to scream as she removes the dressings and the skin that comes with them. Attrition is high among medical professionals who work with burn patients, due to the intense physical and emotional stress of their patients.

Despite the effectiveness of antibiotic creams and gels, the best treatment for the burn patient is the delicate operation that places grafts on the damaged areas. Grafting enables the patient to retain vital body functions, such as heat control, thereby increasing chances for surviving.

A skin bank provides the burn center with grafts either from an unknown donor or from family members, or with pigskin. Patients having no usable skin of their own must rely on the best donor match. An autograft, removed from unburned portions of the patient's body, generally can be fused with other skin areas without rejection. Skin used in a graft can be expanded three times its normal size because of the elastic properties of collagen, the "glue" of connective tissue. Taken from a cadaver, a homograft serves as a bandage, allowing the body to regenerate its own skin. The patient's immunological system usually rejects a homograft after several weeks. Pigskin, which is used for massive burns, is rejected in a week, necessitating frequent replacement.

The graft is rejected when histocompatibility antigens recognize the invading tissue and fight it. Histocompatibility antigens are molecules that differ from one individual to another, each in a special pattern similar to blood type. The antigens are a chemical key to the physician, helping him gauge tissue's response to a graft. Family members, with slightly differing keys, make good donors. An identical twin, sharing the same chemical program, is the best donor for his twin.

Patients who receive pigskin grafts stand the greatest chance of rejection and subsequent in-

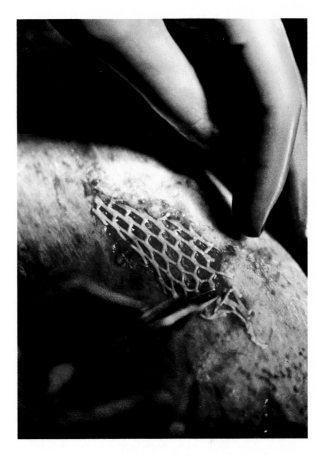

Meshed fabric of skin, the burn patient's own, is stretched over raw flesh and sutured. Before applying the autograft, technicians cut away dead skin and stanch bleeding. To avoid excessive weight loss — and slower healing — a severely burned patient must consume up to three times the calories and protein a healthy person requires.

Artificial skin of collagen fabricated from animal tissue and bonded to a silicone film is applied to third-degree burns. After about twenty days, doctors peel off the silicone and stitch on the meshed autograft.

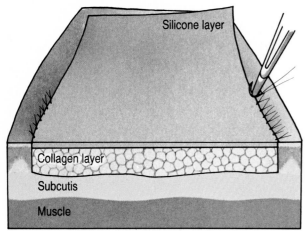

Application of artificial skin to wound

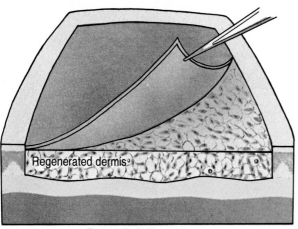

Removal of silicone layer

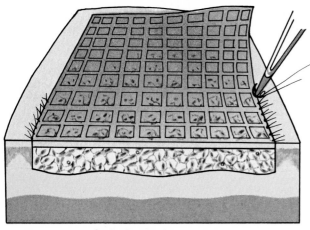

Graft of patient's own skin

fection. Immunosuppressives such as cortisone prolong the life of the graft but make the patient more susceptible to infection. Burn patients can die weeks and months after the burn incident.

Artificial Skin

The drawbacks of donor grafts led doctors and engineers at M.I.T. and Massachusetts General Hospital to develop artificial skin that enables the patient to grow his own skin into a synthetic scaffold. The artificial skin consists of two layers. Polysaccharide polymer, a starchy substance from shark cartilage, bonds with fiber collagen from cowhide to form the latticelike inner layer. This adheres to the outer layer of rubberlike silicone plastic. The two-layer artificial skin is applied to the cleaned wound and sutured at the edges. The shield creates a successful environment for proper cellular growth. As the body's enzymes break down the bottom layer, cells migrate into the lower layer and replace it.

Professor Ioannis Yannas of M.I.T. says that the artificial membrane must be large enough to bring the ends of the wound together and supple enough to adhere to the wound's surface to displace air pockets where infection can hide. After an average of twenty days, the upper layer of silicone is peeled off and replaced with patches of the patient's own epidermal cells, a process which may result in less scarring than normal grafting produces. Yannas and John F. Burke, chief of the Massachusetts General Hospital burn center, have added a new wrinkle to their skin substitute — applying burned areas with artificial skin that has been seeded with basal skin cells taken from the patient. The basal cells regenerate the epidermis beneath the silicone layer, thus eliminating the need for further grafts. They have successfully tested the technique on guinea pigs and expect trials on human burn patients soon. According to Yannas, "Our solution to skin burns suggests that similar procedures can repair other damaged tissues, such as internal organs, without forming scar tissue." By permitting biological interaction with live tissue, the synthetic membrane stimulates cell growth in the proper chemical balance. Appropriately designed biodegradable templates might be used to regenerate

Ioannis Yannas

A Second Skin for Burns

Substances extracted from shark cartilage and cowhide connective tissue covered by a silicone membrane form a synthetic skin that promises new hope for severe burn victims. As thin as a paper towel, the biodegradable substitute has been hailed as a momentous medical advance that is sure to save thousands of lives.

Physical chemist Ioannis V. Yannas heads the M.I.T. laboratory that developed the synthetic skin. Collaborating with John F. Burke, chief of the Massachusetts General Hospital Trauma Services, he has spent more than a decade looking for a way to cover severely burned skin so that it can heal itself without any further treatment. "We don't want to use the patient's own skin at all," he explains.

Until now, doctors have been forced to use the skins of animals and cadavers to cover severe burns. Patients' immune systems react violently to both measures, complicating the attempts to help the body heal itself. The Yannas and Burke design is based on skin's structure, with the silicone layer corresponding to the surface epidermis and the fibrous layer to the deeper dermis. The synthetic membrane triggers no rejection reaction. Keeping vital fluids in and lethal bacteria

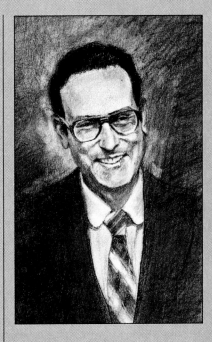

out, it acts like real skin, a temporary trellis to protect the natural healing process. Nerve cells grow slowly into the first layer of the membrane, allowing the patient to actually feel heat and cold.

After a few weeks, the organic part of the membrane dissolves and the plastic is peeled off, revealing a yellow-to-red neodermis populated with living cells and vessels. Doctors then strip extremely thin patches of skin from healthy areas of the patient's body and expand these over the new dermis. The graft heals to normal skin thickness within two weeks.

The success of the treatment has been excellent, with the wounds accepting nearly 100 percent of the artificial skin. Yannas's laboratory can produce about ten square feet of the skin in a few days, or enough to treat a patient burned over 50 percent of his body. Commercial production is on the horizon but Yannas is already at work on an even more effective synthetic skin.

Working with guinea pigs, Yannas has removed basal cells below the skin and used them to "seed" the inner layer of the fabricated skin. Unlike an inert bandage, this enriched sample interacts with the body. It has worked flawlessly. "New and apparently functional skin was generated in less than four weeks," Yannas reported.

Unlocking and putting to use the secrets of tissue regeneration were long thought to be unattainable. The same technique might one day be used to regenerate damaged sections of organs.

The work of Yannas and his colleagues will without doubt inspire new advances in the fight against the horrors of burned flesh. "Artificial skin will go through many forms," says one observer of Yannas's work. "What we have seen today may be just an early stage of the final product."

*This profile of a patient with a
rebuilt nose illustrated Italian
surgeon Gasparo Tagliacozzi's* De
Curtorum Chirurgia, *published in
1597. An innovative thinker, he
borrowed skin from elsewhere on the
patient's body for the reconstruction.*

segments of other tissues that have been lost or
damaged by disease or injury.

One of the first success stories with artificial
skin involved Mark Walsh, a twenty-five-year-
old electrician. Burned over 80 percent of his
body, his prognosis was grim. Under the care of
Burke and Yannas, he responded to treatment
and survived his critical injury. He went home
"feeling great" two months after the accident.

Doctors who operated on Mark Walsh used
both his own skin and the artificial skin. Burke
applied eight square feet of artificial skin on the
neck, chest, abdomen and arms. The scars he will
live with will not be dramatic. "He will be able to
function in society without everybody knowing
that he's scarred, because his face and hands will
be very presentable."

The ability of the surgeon to refashion and re-
shape parts of the body disfigured by disease or
injury resulted in the specialty of plastic surgery.
Plastic derives from the Greek *plastikos,* meaning
"fit for molding," an apt description of plastic
surgery's function. The technique expanded into
the field of cosmetic surgery — the reshaping of
natural disfigurements. Wizards of the scalpel
routinely repair mismatched eyes and ears, bob
noses that are too long and add hair to a balding
head. They also relieve the discomfort of stooped
shoulders by reducing the size of breasts that are
too large.

Radical mastectomy combines the removal of
the breast with some of the pectoral muscles and
the lymph nodes under the arm. Traditionally,
doctors advised a woman who had undergone
breast surgery to get a prosthesis. Today, women
are encouraged to consider reconstructive surgery. Replacement of the breast restores confi-
dence and lessens the sense of loss. As one
surgeon said, "Compared to a natural, normal
breast, the breast produced by postmastectomy
reconstruction is less than perfect," but "nothing
short of a miracle."

An ancient art, plastic surgery was practiced in
India 3,000 years ago to repair noses and ear lobes
injured in battle. Chinese physicians in the third
century reconstructed cleft lips. In 1597, Gasparo
Tagliacozzi of Bologna published the first book
on plastic surgery, *De Curtorum Chirurgia.* In it he

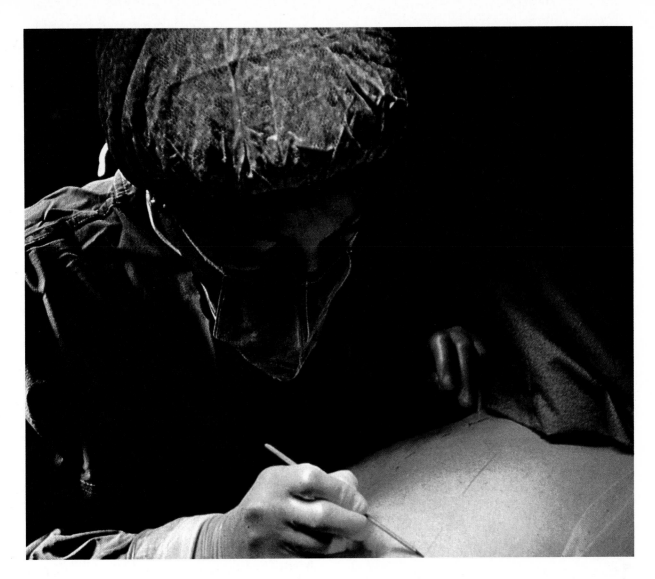

described nasal reconstruction using arm flaps. Because it "meddled with the will of God," the Church opposed his work. But Tagliacozzi himself declared, "We restore, repair and make whole those parts of the face which nature has given but which fortune has taken away, not so much that they may delight the eye, but that they may buoy up the spirit and help the mind of the afflicted."

Sir Harold Gillies, the father of modern plastic surgery, published *Plastic Surgery of the Face* in response to the serious facial injuries suffered by soldiers fighting in the trenches of World War I. Today, plastic surgery has expanded into other fields — ophthalmology, otolaryngology, orthopedics and urology — thanks to the creation of instruments that can deal with the microscopic.

For nearly nine hours, in December of 1981, plastic surgeons in Philadelphia labored to reconstruct the face of a woman horribly deformed by neurofibromatosis. The growths covered her head and scalp in rough lumps and folds. A realist, the woman told a reporter, "I know I am not going to look like Farrah Fawcett-Majors. . . . I would elect to have this surgery even if it gave me only one percent improvement."

Under chief surgeon Linton Whitaker, the Philadelphia doctors cut away massive chunks of bulging flesh, lifting the skin to excise the roots of the growths. The woman's nasal bones had been wrecked by the disease. The surgeons made new ones, using parts of her ribs. When the bandages and dressings were unwrapped three days later, she had a new face. Observers were stunned by the improvement. Plastic surgery had gained a victory, however incomplete, against the most disfiguring of diseases. John Merrick, the Elephant Man, who had once been displayed as a sideshow freak, might be pleased by the progress we have made.

Glossary

acne an inflammatory disease of the hair follicle and sebaceous gland; the common variety is called acne vulgaris.

acupuncture a traditional Chinese method of medical therapy and anesthesia using fine needles to puncture the skin at specific points on the body.

acyclovir a drug used in the initial outbreak of herpes that works by interfering with the ability of the herpes virus to reproduce.

adrenal glands two glands, one above each kidney, that secrete hormones, epinephrine and other substances.

albinism a genetically inherited condition in which the individual is unable to form melanin, resulting in unpigmented skin, hair and eyes. Albinos are highly sensitive to light.

alopecia areata a disease of the face and scalp marked by patchy hair loss.

androgenetic alopecia *see* male-pattern baldness.

anthropometry the study of the size, weight and proportions of the human body, used in anthropology and occasionally in criminology.

apocrine gland a gland that contributes part of its cellular substance to its secretion, such as certain axillary and genital sweat glands.

arrector pili a small smooth muscle of the skin attached to a hair follicle which contracts and pulls the hair erect in response to cold and other stimuli.

arteriovenous anastomosis a connection between an artery and a vein that serves to bypass a bed of capillaries.

autograft a tissue graft from one part of a person's body to another part.

axillary of or relating to the armpit.

Bacchic of or relating to Bacchus, Greek mythology's god of the vineyard and wine.

bacillus any rod-shaped bacterium, especially of the genus *Bacillus*; pl. bacilli.

basal cell cancer malignant growth of the cells in the deepest layer of the epidermis; also called basaloma and basal cell carcinoma.

basal the deepest layer of the epidermis, consisting of a single row of columnar or cuboidal cells; also called the *stratum basale*.

benzoyl peroxide a crystalline substance that induces skin peeling to help clear hair follicles clogged by common acne.

benzyl benzoate the main ingredient in a lotion used to kill scabies mites.

bertillonage *see* anthropometry.

biofeedback the use of electronic equipment to teach subjects how to regulate physical processes normally thought beyond conscious control.

biopsy the removal and examination of tissue from the living body to establish a diagnosis.

bitumen hydrocarbon substances such as tar and pitch derived from coal and oil and used today to seal roofs and roads.

body painting the use of paint to decorate the body symbolically or cosmetically for ritual or celebration.

bubo an inflamed and enlarged lymph node, especially in the groin or axillary region, caused by syphilis, tuberculosis, plague and other diseases; the source of the name bubonic plague.

carcinogen any cancer-causing substance.

cerebellum an oval-shaped portion of the brain situated above the medulla and beneath the cerebrum, concerned with equilibrium and movement.

chicken pox *see* varicella.

clindamycin an antibiotic used against bacteria and parasites.

collagen a protein, and the main supportive constituent of bone, cartilage, connective tissue and skin.

comedo a plug of dried sebaceous and keratinous material in a hair follicle, commonly called a blackhead.

conduction the transmission of energy from one point to another.

Condylomata acuminata a variety of infectious wart with a treelike structure found in moist regions of the skin, particularly around the genitals.

congenital ectodermal defect an uncommon hereditary condition characterized by an absence of sweat glands and malformed teeth and hair; also known as ectodermal dysplasia.

connective tissue a general term for tissue that binds together and supports various parts of the body; consists largely of collagen.

contact dermatitis an acute, allergic inflammation of the skin; usually a delayed reaction caused by contact with a substance to which a person has developed an allergic sensitivity.

convection the transfer of heat in liquids or gases by the movement of heated particles.

corium *see* dermis.

corneal the outermost layer of the epidermis, consisting of flat, hardened, keratinized cells; also called the *stratum corneum*.

corpuscle a term applied to any minute mass, body or particle.

cortex the middle layer of the hair, surrounding the medulla and surrounded by the cuticle.

corticosteroid any of the hormones produced by the cortex of the adrenal gland, or its synthetic substitute; often used to control inflammation and to suppress the immune system.

Corynebacterium acnes a bacterium of the skin usually found in acne lesions.

cosmetics any concoction or procedure applied to the skin or hair for purposes of beautification.

cosmetic surgery the alteration of superficial features for the purpose of beautification.

couvade the practice in some cultures of a husband taking to bed when his wife experiences labor and childbirth.

cowpox a mild disease of milk cows, caused by the vaccinia virus, also called vaccinia; the source of the smallpox vaccine for man.

croup a term commonly describing any kind of spasm or disease-related obstruction of the larynx, marked by hoarseness and a barking cough.

Crow a tribe of American Indians whose original territory ranged between the Platte and Yellowstone rivers in what is now Wyoming.

cryosurgery the use of extremely low temperatures in surgery.

cutaneous of or relating to the skin.

cuticle the outermost layer of a hair.

cystic acne a severe form of acne marked by abnormally large cysts containing sebum and keratinized cells.

cystic fibrosis a hereditary disorder of the exocrine system marked by obstruction of the pancreatic and bile ducts, the bronchi and the intestines.

dapsone an antibacterial compound used in the treatment of leprosy and tuberculosis.

Demodex folliculorum a harmless mite that lives in hair follicles of the face and nose.

dermabrasion a procedure that involves freezing the skin and removing layers of the epidermis and dermis with a high-speed diamond wheel; used to remove tattoos and scars from acne and chicken pox.

dermal papillae the small, nipplelike protrusions of the dermis that reach into the epidermis, bringing food and oxygen to the lower layers of epidermal cells.

dermatitis any inflammation of the skin.

dermatitis herpetiformis a chronic skin disorder characterized by eruptions of itchy papules and blisters, mostly on the arms and abdomen.

dermatoglyphics the study of the patterns of ridges on the skin, especially on the palms, soles and fingertips.

dermatology the science of the diagnosis and treatment of diseases of the skin.

dermatosis any disorder of the skin, especially one without inflammation.

dermis the layer of connective tissue under the epidermis containing blood vessels, nerves, hair follicles, sweat glands and sebaceous glands; also called the corium.

digitate wart a wart with fingerlike protrusions growing from its surface.

eccrine gland a sweat gland, a gland that secretes moisture on the surface of the skin primarily to cool the body through evaporation.

eczema a superficial inflamation of the skin causing redness, itching and scales.

elastin a yellowish protein having the ability to stretch and contract; found in the skin and other tissues.

encephalitis an inflammation of the brain.

endogenous pyrogen a naturally occurring substance in the body that produces fever.

endorphins a term used generally to refer to all substances in the body having opiatelike qualities, including beta-endorphins and enkephalins.

enzyme a protein that accelerates or promotes a chemical change in other substances without being changed itself.

epidermis the outermost layer of skin, above the dermis.

epigamic relating to sexual dominance.

epinephrine a hormone produced by the adrenal gland that stimulates heart muscle, increases the amount of blood pumped by the heart, increases blood pressure and affects the body in many other ways; often called adrenalin.

erythroderma a term describing abnormal redness of the skin, generally over much or all of the body.

erythromycin a widely used antibiotic produced by a variety of the bacterium *Streptomyces erythreus*.

estrogen a general term for female sex hormones that are responsible for secondary female sex characteristics.

eumelanin one of the body's two forms of melanin. The pigment produces shades of brown and black and colors the skin, hair and eyes.

exocrine system the glands that empty their secretions into the body or onto the surface of the skin through a duct, such as an eccrine gland.

fibroblasts connective tissue cells that differentiate into the various kinds of

cells that make collagen, elastin, tendons and other varieties of connective tissue.

filiform wart a wart with threadlike protrusions on its surface.

flexural psoriasis psoriasis occuring mainly at points where the skin folds, such as the elbow or other joints.

formaldehyde a colorless gas that can be used in solution as a preservative and disinfectant.

free nerve endings branched end segments of nerves in the dermis that record sensations, especially pain.

frostbite damage to body tissues exposed to low temperatures.

Galla a pastoral Hamitic people of East Africa.

gamma globulin a substance prepared from blood plasma that includes antibodies and many other components of blood; widely used to combat measles, hepatitis and other diseases.

granular the layer of the epidermis just above the spinous layer, composed of a few rows of cells filled with granules of a precursor of keratin.

guttate psoriasis a variety of psoriasis characterized by small, distinct patches of red, scaly skin.

hair follicle a tunnel-like segment of the epidermis that extends down into the dermis; the structure that produces a hair.

Hansen's disease *see* leprosy.

harijans *see* untouchables.

hemodialyzer a device for removing blood from the body, cleansing it and returning it to the body; also called the artificial kidney.

herpes simplex a viral disease characterized by the appearance of small blisters. Herpes simplex I usually appears near the mouth, herpes simplex II in the genital region.

herpes zoster *see* shingles and varicella.

histamines crystalline compounds that stimulate gastric secretions, dilate blood vessels and constrict smooth muscle, especially in the lungs.

Hodgkin's disease a disorder of the lymphatic tissue characterized by enlargement of the lymph nodes and sometimes accompanied by weight loss, fever and other symptoms.

homograft a tissue graft between individuals of the same species.

hyperthermia abnormally elevated body temperature.

hypertrichosis excessive hair growth.

hypothalamus a structure lying deep in the brain concerned with hormone secretions, body temperature, water balance and other internal conditions of the body.

hypothermia abnormally low body temperature.

Iggo dome receptors configurations of Merkel's disks arranged into bundles.

impetigo a contagious infection of the skin caused by streptococcal and staphyloccal bacteria, marked by small pustules that rapidly cluster into larger blisters.

impetigo herpetiformis a rare and sometimes fatal disease afflicting pregnant women.

interferon small proteins produced in cells that inhibit the multiplication of viruses.

irezumi the Japanese art of tattooing producing traditional patterns that cover most of the body.

keloid scar tissue that covers a wound with more cells than were originally present forming a bulge of tissue.

keratin a tough protein which is the major constituent of skin, hair and nails.

keratinocytes the variety of epidermal cell that manufactures keratin.

Krause end bulbs oval-shaped receptors in the epidermis believed to detect heat, cold and pressure.

Langerhans cell a phagocytic cell in the epidermis that devours bacteria or other foreign substances that penetrate the outer layers of the epidermis.

lanugo the soft, fine hair covering the body of the fetus.

lentigo a heavily pigmented tan or brown spot on the skin caused by an increased number of melanocytes.

leprosy a chronic, communicable disease marked by lesions of the skin and mucous membranes; may also involve periphral nervous tissue and bone.

lesion any wound, sore or tissue damage caused by injury or disease.

lipocytes a connective tissue cell which stores fat; a fat cell.

louse any of several varieties of parasitic insects that infest the skin and hair of mammals.

lunula the small, pale crescent at the root of the nail.

lupus a general term to describe any of several related diseases, especially of the skin and mucous membranes, usually marked by brown or red skin lesions.

Lyme disease a disease which begins as a rash and leads to fever, vomiting, stiffness and inflammation; spread by ticks.

macule a flat, discolored spot on the skin, such as a freckle.

Maenads Greek mythology's female members of Dionysus's orgiastic cult.

male-pattern baldness common baldness; also called androgenetic alopecia.

Malphigian a collective term for the basal, spinous and granular layers of the epidermis; the part of the skin whose cells undergo cell division causing the skin to replace lost cells continuously; also called the *stratum germinativum.*

mastectomy the surgical removal of the breast.

mastopexy a surgical treatment to correct a pendulous breast.

medulla the central core of a hair.

Meissner's corpuscles egg-shaped receptors located between the dermis and epidermis that inform the brain exactly where the skin is touched.

melanin the dark pigment of the hair, skin and eye.

melanocyte a cell that synthesizes melanin.

melanoma a tumor consisting of cells pigmented with melanin.

melanosomes granules of melanin inside melanocytes.

meningitis inflammation of the meninges, the membranes that cover the brain and spinal column.

mercaptan N-acetyl cysteine a chemical used experimentally to remove dead tissue from burn wounds.

Merkel's disks oval-shaped receptors located in the epidermis thought to inform the brain of continuous touch on an area of the skin.

methotrexate an antimetabolic drug sometimes used in severe psoriasis which acts by inhibiting acid production necessary for cellular reproduction.

minoxidil a drug used to treat high blood pressure that may cause the growth of hair as a side effect.

morphine an addictive derivative of opium used in medicine as an anesthetic and a sedative.

moxibustion a method of producing a mild skin irritation to relieve a deeper inflammation; involves the combustion of a small tuft of material, usually from the moxa plant, placed on or just over the skin.

muisaks the avenging spirits of victims of Jivaro head shrinkers.

mummy the body of a person or an animal preserved by embalming; from the Arabic *mumiya,* the oil-based wax used by the ancient Egyptians in their embalming process.

Mycobacterium leprae the bacterium that causes leprosy.

naloxone a drug that blocks the effects of endorphins and opiates.

natron a sodium carbonate salt used by the ancient Egyptians in embalming.

neurofibromatosis a genetically transmitted disorder of the nervous system, bones, muscles and skin resulting in soft tumors, especially on the skin.

neuron the basic conducting unit of the nervous system, also called a nerve cell, consisting of a cell body and threadlike projections that conduct electrical impulses.

neurotransmitter   one of approximately thirty chemical messengers that transmit impulses between neurons.

nevus   a skin lesion that can take many forms — smooth or rough, raised or flat, regularly or irregularly shaped, colored or not. Having no external causes, nevi are assumed to be inherited.

Nuba   a black African tribe inhabiting the southern Sudan.

O-kee-pa   a religious ceremony of the Mandan Indians of North America that involves hoisting participants off the ground by wooden splints piercing the skin of their chests and backs.

ophthalmology   the specialty of medicine concerned with the function, anatomy and diseases of the eye.

opiates   any of the family of sleep-inducing or pain-killing drugs derived from two species of *Papaver*, the poppy plant, including morphine, codeine, paperavine and thebaine.

ornatrix   handmaidens attending women in their boudoir in ancient Rome.

orthopedics   the medical specialty concerned with the study and treatment, often surgical, of the skeletal system and associated organs.

otolaryngology   the medical specialty encompassing the study and treatment of the ear, nose and throat.

ozone   a pale, blue gas that filters ultraviolet radiation from the atmosphere.

PABA   para-amniobenzoic acid; a sun-screening agent that absorbs ultraviolet radiation.

Pacinian corpuscles   fast-reacting, onion-shaped receptors located in the dermis and believed to provide instant information about where we move.

palmist   one who practices palmistry.

palmistry   the practice of reading the future and personality in the patterns of wrinkles in the palm of the hand; also called chiromancy.

papilla   nipplelike projections of the dermis that press into the epidermis; a papilla nourishes every hair follicle.

papillary layer   the upper layer of the dermis, where the dermis meets the epidermis, marked by small protusions, the papillae, that reach into the epidermis.

papillary ridges   rows of papillae that protrude up from the dermis into the epidermis; responsible for fingerprints and other patterns on the skin of the hands, feet and body.

parfumeur   a manufacturer or vendor of cosmetics.

phaeomelanin   one of the two forms of melanin in man. Phaeomelanin is the pigment of red hair.

phagocytic   relating to cells which engulf and digest other cells or debris. From the Greek *phagein*, "to eat."

phantom limb   the perception of receiving sensations from a limb or portion of a limb that has been amputated.

pharmacology   the science of the effects, uses and composition of drugs.

physiognomy   the art of divining a person's future and judging character from signs in facial features.

pigment   any naturally occuring or fabricated substance that gives color, especially to the skin.

piloerection   hair standing on end.

pituitary gland   the small endocrine gland at the base of the brain whose excretions control growth, metabolism and maturation.

Pityrosporum ovale   yeastlike fungi that live on the face and scalp and are nonpathogenic.

placebo   a nonactive substance presented to a patient to satisfy a psychological need for medicine.

plantar wart   a wart on the sole of the foot.

porphyria   an abnormal increase of production of formation of porphyrin — one of the building blocks of respiratory pigments — in the blood, bone marrow and other tissues.

prostaglandins   a group of naturally produced fatty acids that stimulate the contraction of smooth muscle.

prosthesis   any artificial device used to replace a lost part of the body.

psoralens   derivatives of certain plants that cause phototoxic dermatitis when in contact with skin that has been exposed to sunlight.

psoriasis   a hereditary skin disease which produces red sores covered with silver scales found usually on the scalp, knees and elbows.

Pseudomonas   a genus of bacteria with tail-like flagella that can propel them through air, water, soil and sewage. The species *aeruginosa* can cause infections in burns.

Reins barrier   a thin structure that protects epidermal cells from dehydration.

reticular layer   the lower layer of the dermis, a tough web of collagen and elastin.

rhinoscleroma   a disease of the skin in which sensitive patches form around the nose and nasopharynx.

rickets   a disease of children that prevents normal bone formation, caused by a deficiency of vitamin D, resulting in soft and often deformed bones.

Rickettsia prowazeki   a parasitic bacterium that causes typhus, transmitted to humans by lice.

ringworm   any of several skin diseases caused by fungi and characterized by circular, itchy patches on the skin.

rubella   German measles; a short-lived, contagious viral disease causing skin eruptions; most dangerous to women in their first weeks of pregnancy.

rubeola   measles, red eruptions on the skin caused by a virus and accompanied by swelling of the mucous membrane and fever.

Ruffini endings   receptors located in the epidermis that scientists believe detect heat, cold and pressure.

scabies   burrows in the skin caused by the itch mite which become inflamed and are often attended by eczema.

scalping   the removal of a defeated enemy's scalp and hair as a trophy and as a means to capture spiritual strength.

scarification   the art of decorating the body with geometric scars, practiced mainly in Africa.

scleroderma the thickening and hardening of the skin caused by disease.

scrofula a tubercular infection of the lymph nodes of the neck, usually in children, caused by the bacterium *Mycobacterium bovis*. For several centuries in England and France, the touch of the king was thought to cure scrofula.

Scythians members of an ancient nomadic tribe that inhabited parts of southeastern Europe and southern Asia.

sebaceous gland a gland beneath the skin that secretes sebum into the hair follicle.

seborrhea a disorder of the sebaceous gland that causes excessive secretion of sebum resulting in scales or an oily coating on the skin.

sebum a semifluid substance secreted by the subaceous glands composed of waxes, fatty acids, cholesterol and debris from skin cells.

seratonin a substance produced in the body that constricts blood vessels.

set point the body's normal temperature, varying from individual to individual but averaging 98.6° F.; akin to the setting on a thermostat, the set point represents the center of the body's temperature balance.

shingles herpes zoster; painful eruptions of vesicles following nerve paths on one side of the body caused by the varicella-zoster virus, which also causes chicken pox.

silicone a broad term for polymers that are water-repellent and physiologically inert; used as coatings for adhesives and electrical wiring, and for the construction of artificial body parts.

silver sulfadiazine a silver solution used in place of silver nitrate for treatment of burns.

smooth muscle nonstriated muscle not under voluntary control, such as the muscles of the intestines and blood vessels, and the arrector pili muscles that attach to hair follicles.

soap a concoction of sodium salts derived from the acids of fats and oils and used for cleaning.

spinous the middle layer of the epidermis, between the basal and granular layers; also called the *stratum spinosum*.

squamous cell a flat, scalelike cell of the epithelium, such as a cell lining the digestive tract or a cell of the outer layers of the skin.

Staphylococcus aureus a species of microorganisms that group in clusters and cause pus-discharging sores on the skin, including boils, carbuncles and abscesses.

stratum basale *see* basal.

stratum corneum *see* corneal.

stratum germinativum *see* Malphigian.

stratum granulosum *see* granular.

stratum spinosum *see* spinous.

subcutis the flexible, fatty and fibrous tissue beneath the skin.

sulfonamides sulfa drugs; used to fight bacteria.

sulfone any of several compounds that contain two hydrocarbons connected to a sulfur-dioxide molecule; used to suppress the growth of bacteria.

syphilis a sexually transmitted disease that progresses from chancres to ulcers and finally to general paresis.

tattoo the placing of pigments between the dermis and epidermis to stain the skin for permanent decoration.

terminal hair visible, pigmented hair, like the hair of the scalp; also called mature hair.

testosterone the principle steroid hormone produced in men; responsible for secondary sex characteristics.

tetracycline an antibiotic with wide-ranging applications produced from mold cultures of *Streptomyces* bacteria or made synthetically.

thalamus the relay center of the brain for sensory impulses.

thermoreceptor any of a variety of nerve endings that register and relay changes in temperature.

13-cis retinoic acid a derivative of vitamin A used to treat cystic acne.

tonsure a hair style consisting of a horseshoe or halo of hair around a bald patch on the crown of the head; worn for centuries by priests and monks as a symbol of humility.

transcutaneous nerve stimulator a portable, battery-operated device that sends electrical impulses through the skin, bringing relief from pain.

trephination any surgery involving the removal of a disk of bone from the skull.

trephine a surgical tool designed and used for cutting out disks of bone or tissue, usually from the skull.

tsanta the shrunken head trophy sought for centuries by the Jivaro warriors of the Andes rain forests of South America.

typhus an infectious fever caused by *Rickettsia* with a symptomatic rash.

tyrosinase the enzyme in body tissue that converts tyrosine into melanin.

untouchables members of the Sudra caste, the lowest level of the Hindu caste system in India; also called *harijans*. Untouchables are considered unclean and their touch is believed to pollute members of higher castes.

urology the branch of medicine that specializes in the study and treatment of the urogenital tract.

urticaria hives; itchy eruptions on the skin brought on by sensitivity to drugs, food and emotional factors.

varicella chicken pox; a contagious childhood disease caused by the varicella-zoster virus, which also causes shingles. Its symptoms are eruptions on the skin, and fever.

variolation inoculation for smallpox.

vellus lightly pigmented, nearly invisible hair that covers the body.

vibrissae sensory hairs, such as the whiskers on a dog.

vitiligo white patches on the skin of the face, neck, hands, thighs and stomach, caused by an absence of melanin.

wart a rough outgrowth of the skin usually caused by a virus.

Yersinia pestis the species of bacterium responsible for bubonic plague; previously called *Pasteurella pestis*.

Yersin's serum antiplague serum developed by Swiss bacteriologist Alexandre E. J. Yersin (1863-1943).

Zomax a new, nonaddictive drug for the treatment of pain.

Illustration Credits

The Body's Frontier
6, London Scientific Fotos.

The Way of All Flesh
8, Malcolm Kirk/Peter Arnold, Inc. 10, The Granger Collection, New York. 11, *Jason with the Golden Fleece* by Peter Paul Rubens, The Granger Collection, New York. 12, The University Museum, University of Pennsylvania. 13, National Museum of American Art, Smithsonian Institution. 14, Benarbter Frauenrucken/ ZEFA. 15, The Granger Collection, New York. 16, George Rodger/Magnum. 17, Walter Firmo/Black Star. 18, Angelo Giampiccolo/Black Star. 19, (top) Bruno Barbey/Magnum (bottom) Bert Miller/ Black Star. 20, Auckland City Art Gallery, New Zealand. 21, Lyle Tuttle Collection. 22, D. Baglin/ZEFA. 23, Peter and Georgina Bowater/The Image Bank. 24, (top) The Brooklyn Museum, Charles Edwin Wilbour Fund (bottom) The Granger Collection, New York. 24-25, Editorial Photocolor Archives, Inc. 27, *Portrait of an Elizabethan Lady,* The Bodleian Library. 28, *Nell Gwyn* by Sir Peter Lely, The Granger Collection, New York. 29, Editorial Photocolor Archives. 30, *The Bather of Valpinçon* by J.A.D. Ingres, The Granger Collection, New York. 31, From the Art Collection of the Folger Shakespeare Library. 32, Shogun Gallery, Washington, DC. 33, (left) The Cleveland Museum of Art, Edward L. Whittemore Fund (right) The Granger Collection, New York. 34, *Napoleon in His Study* by Jacques-Louis David, National Gallery of Art, Washington, DC, Samuel H. Kress Collection. 36, Historical Collections, College of Physicians of Philadelphia. 37, National Library of Medicine.

A Woven Mantle
38, Detail ("L'Odorat") from the *Lady and the Unicorn* tapestry, The Granger Collection, New York. 40, From *Tissues and Organs: A Text Atlas of Scanning Electron Microscopy* by Richard G. Kessel and Randy H. Kardon, © 1979 W. H. Freeman & Co. 41, **Thomas B. Allen.** 42, **Dan Sherbo.** 43, Manfred Kage/Peter Arnold, Inc. 44, Biophoto Associates/ Paul Wheater. 45, **Modern Artz.** 46, (top) Bob Stern/International Stock Photography (bottom) S. Weiss/Photo Researchers. 47, C.M. Papa, M.D. © 1970. 48, (top) Biophoto Associates (bottom) National Library of Medicine. 49, Skip Brown. Foldout, (outside) National Library of Medicine (inside) **Carol Donner.** 50, **Thomas B. Allen.** 51, National Library of Medicine. 53, Skip Brown. 54, *Satan Smiting Job with Sore Boils* by William Blake, The Granger Collection, New York. 55, Lennart Nilsson from his book *Behold Man,* published in the U.S. by Little, Brown & Co., Boston. 56, Larry Burrows, *Life,* © Time Inc. 57, Manfred Kage/Peter Arnold, Inc. 58, Historical Collections, College of Physicians of Philadelphia. 59, The Granger Collection, New York. 60, The Bettmann Archive. 61, C. James Webb.

Barrier to the World
62, Manfred Kage/Peter Arnold, Inc. 64, Howard Sochurek. 65, **Modern Artz.** 66, S. M. Estvanik/FPG. 67, Unilever Research, Port Sunlight, England. 69, The Bettmann Archive. 70-71, David Moore/ Black Star. 71, (right) © D.W. Fawcett; G. Szabo/Photo Researchers. 72, (top) Field Museum of Natural History, Chicago (bottom) Runk/Schoenberger of Grant Heilman Photography. 74-75, Louis Goldman/Photo Researchers. 76, **Modern Artz.** 77, Jonathan Blair/Woodfin Camp, Inc. 78, **Thomas B. Allen.** 79, J.F. Gennaro/Photo Researchers.

Finery on the Fabric
80, *Self-Portrait* by Albrecht Dürer, The Granger Collection, New York. 82, Michael Abbey/Photo Researchers. 83, P. Thurston/The Daily Telegraph Colour Library. 84, *Tissues and Organs: A Text Atlas of Scanning Electron Microscopy* by Richard G. Kessel and Randy H. Kardon, © 1979 W.H. Freeman & Co. 85, **Carol Donner.** 86, (top) Lennart Nilsson from his book *Behold Man,* published in the U.S. by Little, Brown & Co., Boston (bottom) Michael Abbey/Photo Researchers. 87, The Mansell Collection. 88, Manfred Kage/Peter Arnold, Inc. 89, The Granger Collection, New York. 90, Animals Animals/Zig Leszczynski. 91, Courtesy of Lucasfilm Ltd. (LFL) 1980. All rights reserved. 92, *Samson Betrayed by Delilah* by Rembrandt, Scala/Editorial Photocolor Archives. 93, Scala/Editorial Photocolor Archives. 94, Jeff Beaudry/ Editorial Photocolor Archives. 95, BBC Hulton Picture Library. 96, Mary Evans Picture Library. 97, *Portrait of a Lady* by Rogier van der Weyden, National Gallery of Art, Washington, DC, Andrew W. Mellon Collection. 98, The Granger Collection, New York. 99, Editorial Photocolor Archives. 100, Print Collection; Art, Prints and Photographs Division, The New York Public Library, Astor, Lenox and Tilden Foundation. 101, Historical Pictures Service, Inc. 103, Courtesy of Fruitlands Museums, Harvard, MA. 104, The Bettmann Archive. 105, Hiroji Kubota/Magnum. 106, Personality Photos, Inc. 107, (top) John Veltri/Photo Researchers (bottom) Colour Library International. 108, (top) Eve Arnold/Magnum (bottom) Popperfoto Ltd. 109, L.H. Mangino/FPG.

The Human Touch
110, *The Brothers* by Ben Shahn, Hirshhorn Museum and Sculpture Garden, Smithsonian Institution, © Estate of Ben Shahn. 112, University Library of Cambridge, Cambridge, England. 113, Lawrence Marshall. 115, Erich Hartmann/ Magnum. 116, Richard Kalvar/Magnum. 117, René Burri/Magnum. 118, Bernard Wolff/Photo Researchers. 121, David Linton from *Scientific American.* 123, J. Alex Langley/Design Photographers International. 122, The Bettmann Archive. 124, William Harnsen. 125, Micha Bar Am/Magnum. 126, Courtesy of Bakken Library, Minneapolis, MN. 127, Dan McCoy/Rainbow. 128, Editorial Photocolor Archives. 129, Akira Hagihara/Visions.

A Thousand Natural Shocks
130, *The Dead Marat* by Jacques-Louis David, Scala/Editorial Photocolor Archives. 132, Cabinet des Manuscrits, Bibliothèque Royale, Belgium. 133, Ann Ronan Picture Library. 134, **Thomas B. Allen.** 135, Dr. Gerald P. Walsh, Armed Forces Institute of Pathology. 137, Charles Harbutt/Archive. 138, Hal McKusick/Design Photographers International. 139, K.S. Shields, USDA Forest Service, Hamden, Connecticut. 140, (top) Phillip Harrington/The Image Bank (bottom) Painting by Frederick Bertucci; photo by Bernard Edelman. 141, The Granger Collection, New York. 142, Illustration by Donald McKay from *The Adventures of Tom Sawyer* by Mark Twain; illustrations © 1946, renewed 1974 by Grosset & Dunlap, Inc. 143, Darwin Dale. 144, National Library of Medicine. 145, (both) PHOTRI. 147, Ann Ronan Picture Library. 148, (top) P.G. Nunn (bottom) Historical Collections, College of Physicians of Philadelphia. 149, Culver Pictures. 150, Don Carstens. 151, Don Carstens. 152, **Diane Robertson.** 153, **Thomas B. Allen.** 154, The Bettmann Archive. 155, Sebastiao Salgado/ Magnum.

Index

Page numbers in bold type indicate location of illustrations.

A
accidental pattern, 49
acupuncture, 128
Aesculapius, 34
Afro, 107, 108
Agent Orange, 140
albinism, 72
Alibert, J. L. B., 35-36
allergen, 138-141
    chocolate, 138
    strawberries, 138
    mold, 139
    larvae, gypsy moth, 139
    milk, 140
    pollen, 140
    dander, 141
    wool, 141
    feathers, 141
allergy, 20, 131, 138
amino acid, 52
anastomosis, 65-66, **65**
Anatomia Humani Corporis, 51
Angley, Ernest, 111
animal skin, 11
anthropometry, 51, 52
antibiotics, 45, 52, 54, 57, 60, 141, 151
antibody, 141
antigen, 141, *see also* allergen
antihistamine, 141, 142, 143
antiperspirant, 47
Antoinette, Marie, 87, 100
Apollo, 34
arch, 48-49
Aristophanes, 34
armadillo, 39, 136
arrector pili, 65, **65**, 84, **85**
artery, *foldout*, 65
*Artificial Embellishments, or Art's Best
    Directions How to Preserve Beauty or
    Procure It*, 29
artificial skin, 152, **152**, 153, 154
Astruc, Jean, 35
athlete's foot, 58
autograft, 151, 152
autoimmunity, 138, 141

B
Bacchus, 11
bacterium, 11, 27, 43, 44, 45, 46, 54, 56,
    57, 58, 69, 83, 114, 131, 136, 141,
    144, 153
baldness, 87-91, 94, 95, 98
    alopecia areata, 87, 89
    androgenetic alopecia, 89
Bartholomew the Englishman, 133, 135
basal layer, 40, *foldout*, 76, 79
Bateman, Thomas, 35
bath, 30, 34
beard, 58, 94, 95, 96, 98, 99, 102, 103,
    104, 105, 108

beauty spot, 131
Beecher, Henry, 121
benzoyl peroxide, 45
benzyl benzoate, 54
Bernard, Sister Solange, 137
Bernhardt, Sarah, 31
Bertillon, Alphonse, 52
bertillonage, 52
Bidloo, Govard, 51
biodegradable template, 152
biofeedback, 128
biopsy, 136
bite, 131, 142, 143
Black Death, 58, 59
blackhead, 45
Blagden, Sir Charles, 67
blister, 56, 67, 131, 138, 139, 143
blood, 54, 58, 63, 67, 120
blood pressure, 43
blood vessel, 42-43, 66, 67, 84, 85, 119,
    140, 141, 153
body decoration, 9, 13, 15-17, 19-20, 23-
    25
body odor, 47, 54
boil, 54
bone, 43, 46, 67
Boswell, James, 113
Brain, Robert, 16
Brummell, Beau, 30, 103
Burke, John F., 152, 153, 154
burn, 86, 120, 131, 150-52, 153, 154

C
callus, 39, 143
capillary, 35, 41, 42, 58
carcinogen, 78
cartilage, 152, 153
Catherine of Braganza, 29
cell, 40, 42, 43, 44, 48, 54, 56, 57, 64, 71,
    72, 76, 84-85, 87, 142, 145, 152, 153
Charles II, 28, 29
chemical, 23, 86, 120, 121, 138
chigger, 54
chiothetist, *see* hand healer
cholesterol, 43
claw, 40, 81
clitoris, 119
collagen, 42, 43, 138, 151, 152, **152**
comedo, 44, 45, **45**
conduction, 64
Confessions of an English Opium Eater, 122
connective tissue, 40, 84
convection, 64
Convit, Jacinto, 136
core, 48-49
corium, 35, 42, *see also* dermis
corn, 37, 143
corneal layer, 40, 42, *foldout*, 43, 73
corticosteroid, 137, 140, *see also* drug,
    cortisone
cosmetic, 9, 24, 25-26, 28-31, 33, 44, 46
cowpox, 146
crew cut, 105, 107

crime, 49, 50
cryosurgery, 23, 79
cyst, 45

D
Dactylography, 50
Damien, Father, 134
dandruff, 87
David, Jacques Louis, 131
DDT, 60
decay, 11
De Curtorum Chirurgia, 154
Defoe, Daniel, 59
dehydration, 68
Delightes for Ladies, 28
delta, 49
Demodex folliculorum, 54
De Quincey, Thomas, 122
dermabrasion, 45
dermatoglyphics, 48
dermatology, history of, 31, 35, 37
dermis, 23, 39, 42, 43, 45, **45**, *foldout*, 51,
    52, 65, 72, 84, 85, 119, 120, 152, **152**,
    153
desmosome, 40
diet, 31, 34, 44
Dillinger, John, 52
DNA, 57, 143
disk, 16, 17
disease and disorder
    acne, 44-45, 54, 137
        Corynebacterium acnes, 54
        cystic, 45
        vulgaris, 45
    bubonic plague, 58-59
    cancer, 40, 75, 76, 78, 79, 127, 140, 143
    chicken pox, 56, 144-45
    cystic fibrosis, 47
    dermatitis, contact, 138-40
        noninfective, 140
        occupational, 140
    dermatitis herpetiformis, 34, 131
    dysplasia, ectodermal, 146
    eczema, 20, 35, 140
        milk crust, 141
        seborrheic, 141
    encephalitis, 56
    Hansen's disease, *see* disease, leprosy
    herpes simplex I, 56, 141
    herpes simplex II, 56
    herpes zoster, 145
    Hodgkin's disease, 145
    hypertrichosis, 149
    impetigo, 37, 141
    jaundice, 9
    leprosy, 131-33, 134, 135-36
    lupus, 141
    Lyme disease, 144
    measles, 144, 145
        German, 49, 144
    mononucleosis, 56
    neurofibromatosis, 146, 147, 148, 155
    plague, 58-60, 113

pneumonia, 59
porphyria, 148-49
prurigo, 37
psoriasis, 132, 136-38
    flexural, 136
    generalized, 136
    guttate, 136
rhinoscleroma, 37
rubella, 144, *see also* measles, German
rubeola, 144, *see also* measles
scabies, 37, 54
schizophrenia, 115
scleroderma, 138
seborrhea, 44
shingles, 56, 145
smallpox, 9, 145-46
systemic sclerosis, 138
typhus, 60
varicella, 144-45
venereal disease, 143
vitiligo, 132, 138
Donne, John, 26
drug, 63, 131, 135
    acyclovir, 57
    aspirin, 68, 69
    clindamycin, 45
    clotrimazole, 58
    codeine, 122
    cortisone, 137, 142, 152
    dapsone, 136, 137
    erythromycin, 45, 141
    gamma globulin, 144
    griseofulvin, 58
    heroin, 122
    interferon, 69, 145
    mercaptan N-acetyl cysteine, 150
    methotrexate, 137
    miconazole, 58
    Minoxidil, 89
    morphine, 121, 122, 127
    naloxone, 122-23
    silver sulfadiazine, 151
    sulfonamide, 141
    tetraycline, 45, 141
    13-cis retinoic acid, 45
    Zomax, 127
dye, 15

E
Eau Dalibour, 141
elastin, 42
electrosurgery, 79
Elephant Man, The, 147, 148
Elizabeth I, 26, 28, 98
embalming, 10
emotion, 9, 44, 46
endorphin, 122, 127, 128
energy, 43, 66
environment, 44
epidermis, 35, 39, 40, 42, 43, 45, **45**, 47,
    foldout, 72, 76, 83, 84, 85, 119, 136,
    152, 153
epinephrine, 120

erythroderma, 136
estrogen, 45
eumelanin, 71
evaporation, 65, 67, 68
exocrine system, 47
eyebrow, 26, 30, 82, 96
eyelash, 82
eyelid, 39, 66, 82

F
faith healing, 111
fat, 43, 44, 57, 58, 70, 82, 83, 84, 89, 138
fatty acid, 43, 44, 45, 56, 68
Faulds, Henry, 50, 51
feather, 81
fever, 68-69, 111
fibroblast, 42, 43
finger, 113
fingernail, 40, 66, 85, 88, 136
fingerprint, 42, 47-49, 50, 51-52, 53
fingertip, 119
flea, 58, 60
food, 131
foot, 39, 66, 67
formaldehyde, 140
freckle, 28-29, 30, 72, 131
Frey, Maximilian von, 120
frostbite, 67
fungus, 58, 69

G
Galen, 35
Galla, 10
Galton, Sir Francis, 51, 52
gene, 40, 56, 70, 76, 85, 136, 146
Gillies, Sir Harold, 155
Giovanni, Nikki, 7
gland
    adrenal, 120
    apocrine, 46-47, 83, *see also* sweat
    eccrine, 46-47, 49, *foldout, see also* sweat
    sebaceous, 35, 42, 43, 44, **45**, *foldout*, 54,
        84, **85**
Goeckerman treatment, 137
Gonzalez, Ernesto, 138
graft, 150-52, **152**, 153
granular layer, 40, *foldout*
Grateau, Marcel, 102-03
graying, 86, 87
Grew, Nehemiah, 51, 52
Gwyn, Nell, 28, 29

H
hair
    axillary, 82, 83
    coloring, 86, 95
    epigamic growth, 83
    follicle, 40, 43, 44, **45**, *foldout*, 54, 82, 83,
        84, 85, 86, 88, 91
    lanugo, 83
    loss of, 89
    magical power, 92-93
    pubic, 83

symbolism of, 82, 91
    transplant, 90-91
    vellus, 83
hairdresser, 100, 102, 103, 107
hair weaving, 89-90
Hall, Edward, 116
hand, 39, 66, 67, 131, 139
hand healer, 113
Hansen, G. Armauer, 135
head shrinking, 12
heat stroke, 68
Hebra, Ferdinand von, 37
Heflin, Richard, 115
hemodialyzer, 67
Henley, Nancy, 117
Henry, Sir Edward, 52
Hercules, 11
Herodotus, 12
herpes virus, 56-57, 141
Herschel, Sir William J., 50
Hetepheres, Queen, 26
Hippocrates, 35
histamine, 120, 139
histocompatibility antigen, 151
hives, 138-39, 143
Hollender, Marc, 115
homograft, 151, **152**
hoof, 40, 81
Hôpital Saint-Louis, 35, 37
hormone, 45, 58, 83, 89
horn, 40, 81
hot tub, 56
hyperthermia, 68
hypnosis, 128, 142
hypothalamus, 47, 64, 65, 68
hypothermia, 66-67

I
Iggo, Ainsley, 120
Iggo dome receptor, 119
immunity, 40, 58, 132, 135, 137, 144, 146,
    151, 153
immunosuppressive, 152
infection, 54, 56, 57, 58, 69, 141
inflammation, 35, **45**
Ingres, Jean Auguste Dominique, 30
inoculation, 136
insulation, 43, 64, 82
integument, 39
interstitial fluid, 65
itch, 54, 58, 136, 138, 139, 141, 145

J
Jeamson, Thomas, 29
Jenner, Edward, 146
Jivaro, *see* head shrinking
Johnson, Samuel, 113-14
Journal of the Plague Year, A, 59

K
Keller, Helen, 112
keloid, 86
keratin, 40, 43, 75, 85, 88

keratinocyte, 40, 43
kiss, 116, 117
Krause end bulb, 119-20

L

Langerhans cell, 40
Langer's lines, 42, **42**, 43
Langtry, Lillie, 31
laser, 23
lazaretto, 133
lazarhouse, *see* lazaretto
Leeuwenhoek, Anton van, 52
legends about skin, 9-10
Le Moyne, Jacques, 13
lentigines, senile, 131
leper, 131-33, 134, 135-36
leprosarium, 133, 134
Lewis, Sinclair, 112
lip, 16, 17, 26, 28, 31, 65, 66, 105, 119
lip disk, 16, 17
lipid, 43
lipocyte, 43
liver spot, *see* lentigines, senile
loop, 48, 49
Lorry, Antoine Charles, 35
Louis XIV, 98-99, 100
louse, 35, 60-61, 59, 60, 61
lovelock, 29, 99
lunula, 85
lymph, 20, 42, 141, 154

M

Macaroni, 100, 101-02
macule, 131
Maenads, 11
make-up, 19, 25-26, 28-31, 33, *see also*
    cosmetic
Malpighi, Marcello, 35, 40, 41, 51
Manson, Sir Patrick, 135
mastectomy, 154
mastopexy, 154
masturbation, 45
Mataora, 17, 20
McPherson, Aimee Semple, 112
Medusa, 92, 93
Meissner's corpuscle, *foldout*, 119-20
melanin, 40, 45, 71, 72-73, 75, 76, **76**, 82,
    85, 86
melanocyte, 40, *foldout*, 71, 72, 76, **76**, 85,
    86, 138
melanoma, 79, 131
melanosome, 71, 72, **76**
Melville, Herman, 20
Mercurialis, Hieronymus, 35
Merkel's disk, 119-20
Merrick, Joseph, 147, 148, 155
metabolism, 63, 70-71
Midrash Rabbah, 135
mitosis, 40
Moko, 17, 20
mole, 79, 131, *see also* nevus
Montagu, Ashley, 115, 116, 147
mouse, 136

movie stars, 106
moxibustion, 128
mucous, membrane, 35
muisak, 11
mummification, 10, 11, 17
muscle, 43, 66, 84, 85, **152**
mustache, 94, 102, 104, 105, 108
mycobacterium leprae, 135

N

Napoleon, 34
Nei Ching, 135
nerve, 35, 42, *foldout*, 56, 57, 64, 66, 82, 84,
    85, 119-20, 121, 153
Nessler, Karl, 87, 106
Nestlé, Charles, *see* Nessler, Karl
neurotransmitter, 120, 122
nevus, 131, 146
Nicholas II, Czar, 16
nipple, 26, 46, 119
nit, 61
Nuba, 15, 25
nucleus, 42, 82, 145
Nuvarahu, 17

O

oil, 43, 63, 84, 85, 95, 103, 139
    Macassar, 103
Olga, Queen, 16
oral contraceptive, 89
ornatrix, 26
Oscar, King, 16
Osler, Sir William, 69
Ovid, 26
oxygen, 54, 67

P

Pacinian corpuscle, *foldout*, 119-20, 121
pain, 15, 90, 120-23
    aching, 121
    burning, 121
    chronic, 127
    pricking, 121
    and religion, 123, 124, 125
painkiller, 121-23
paint, 9, 15, 17, 19, 26
palm, 39, 42, 119, 139
Palmer, Joseph, 103-104
papaya enzyme, 143
papilla, 41, 42, 47-48, *foldout*, 51, 84, 85
para-aminobenzoic acid (PABA), 79
penis, 119
perfume, 26, 29, 46, 47, 95, 117
permanent wave, 86, 87
Peter the Great, 98, 99
phaeomelanin, 71
phantom limb, 126
pheromone, 46
pigskin graft, 151
piloerection, 66
pimple, 30, 45
Pitanguy, Ivo, 154
Pityrosporum ovale, 57

plastic surgery, 46, 154-55
Plastic Surgery of the Face,
Platt, Sir Hugh, 28-29
Pliny the Elder, 16
poison ivy, 138, 139-40
polymer hydrogel, 151
polysaccharide, 152
pomade, 99, 100
Pope, Alexander, 30
pore, 63
porphyrin, 148
Pott, Percivall, 78
powder room, 101
premature infants, 114
prostaglandin, 68, 120, 127
protein, 42
Pseudomonas, 56
psoralen, 138, 141
puberty, 44
punk, 109
Purkinje, Johannes Evangelist, 51
pus, **45**
PUVA, 138
pyrogen, endogenous, 68

Q

quarantine, 135
quill, 81

R

radiation, heat, 64
    ultraviolet, 40, 43, 71, 72, 73, 75, 76, 79,
        137, 141
rash, 60, 131, 138-39, 144
receptor, 65, 119-121
Recklinghausen, von, 147
Reins barrier, 42
reticular layer, 42, 43, *foldout*
Rhus, 139-40
Richards, Martin, 114
Rickettsia prowazeki, 60
ringworm, 37, 58
Rochester, Earl of, 29-30
Roundhead, 99
Royal Touch, 112, 113
Ruffini corpuscle, *foldout*
    ending, 119-20

S

Samson, 91-92
scale, 58, 81
scalp, 13, 81, 83, 87, 88-89, 96
scalping, 12, 13
scar, 9, 15, 23, 25, 34, 39, 42, 43, 45, 79,
    142, 145, 149, 152, 154
scarification, 15
Scythian, 12, 13
sebum, 43-44, 45, **45**, 54, 56, 84, *see also*
    gland, sebaceous
serotonin, 120
set point, 63-64, 68
Seurat, Georges, 33
shaving, 104

Shepard, Charles C., 136
shiver, 66, 69
sideburn, 104, 108
side whiskers, 104, *see also* sideburn
silicone, 152, **152**, 153
skin bank, 151
Smith Papyrus, 113
Snyder, Solomon, 122
soap, 29, 30, 31, 84
sole, 39, 42, 131
space, 116-17
Spenser, Edmund, 26
spinous layer, 40, *foldout*
squamous cell, 76, 79
Staphylococcus aureus, 54
Stenson, Niels, 35
steroid, 139
sting, 131, 142, 143
stratum germinativum, 40
stress, 114
stretching, skin, 16
subcutis, 39, 43, **45**, *foldout*, 138, **152**
sulfur, 45, 54
sun, 40, 43, 45, 72-73, 75, 76, 79, 131, 141,
    147, 148-49
sunburn, 76, 79
Suomi, Stephen, 114
Sutherland sisters, 88
Suga, 16
sweat, 35, 42, 43, 46-47, 51, 52, 54, 65, **65**,
    67-68, 82, 83, 146-47, *see also* gland,
    apocrine *and* gland, eccrine

T
Tagliacozzi, Gasparo, 154-55
tanning, 11, 75-76, **76**, 79
taste bud, 41

tattoo, 16-17, 19, 20, 23
    irezumi, 20, 23
    moko, 20
Teit, James, 24
temperature, 9, 43, 47, 63-65, 68, 143
Terry, Ellen, 31
testosterone, 44
thalamus, 121
Theodora, Empress, 25
Thepu, Lady, 24
thermoreceptor, 65, **65**
Thomas, Lewis, 142
Thompsen Indians, 24, 25
tick, 144
Tiv, 15
toenail, 40
tonsure, 95-96
touch
    deprivations of, 114-15
    ethnic reaction to, 116
    power of, 117
transcutaneous nerve stimulator (TNS),
    127
tsanta, 12
tumor, 138, 148
Twain, Mark, 51, 142
Typee, 20
tyrosinase, 72

U
untouchable, 117, 119
urticaria, 138, *see also* hives

V
vaccination, 136, 144
variola major, 145

variolation, 146
vein, *foldout*, 65
vibrissae, 82
virus, 56, 57, 131, 141, 142, 144, 146
vitamin A, 45
vitamin D, 43, 72-73, 75
Vucetich, Juan, 52

W
wart, 131, 142-43
    Condylomata acuminata, 143
    digitate, 143
    filiform, 143
    flat, 143
    plantar, 143
Whitaker, Linton, 155
Whitaker Negroes, 146-47
white blood cell, 69
whorl, 48-49, 51
wig, 87, 89, 93, 94, 96, 98, 99, 101, 102,
    106, 107
Willan, Robert, 35-36
World Health Organization, 136
World I Live In, The, 112
wrinkle, 9, 31, 46, 76

X
X-ray, 45, 72, 89

Y
Yannas, Ioannis, 152, 153, 154
yeast, 54, 57
*Yellow Emporer's Classic of Internal Medicine,
    The*, 128
Yersinia pestis, 58

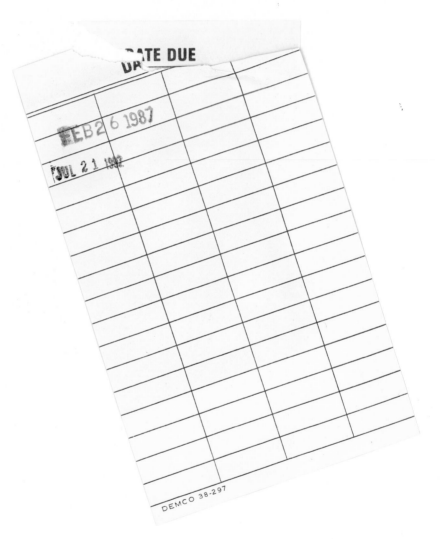

WR100   P742s   10403

Podolsky

The skin

Deleted